Back Pain Matters in Primary Care

Clinical management of back pain in a
healthy and safe environment

Ruth Chambers

Barbara Hawksley

Gill Smith

and

Chris Chambers

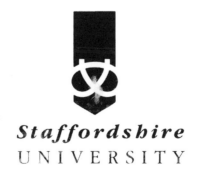

Staffordshire
UNIVERSITY

RADCLIFFE MEDICAL PRESS

© 2001 Staffordshire University
Cartoons © 2001 Martin Davies

Radcliffe Medical Press
18 Marcham Road, Abingdon, Oxon OX14 1AA

British Library Cataloguing in Publication Data

A catalogue record for this book is available from the British Library.

ISBN 1 85775 418 2

Typeset by Joshua Associates Ltd, Oxford
Printed and bound by TJ International Ltd, Padstow, Cornwall

Contents

About the authors

Ruth Chambers has been a GP for 20 years. She has undertaken a wide range of research focusing on stress and the health of doctors, health at work and the quality of healthcare. She is currently the Professor of Primary Care Development at Staffordshire University. Ruth has designed and organised many types of educational initiatives, including distance learning programmes. Recently she has developed a keen interest in working with GPs, nurses and others in primary care around clinical governance and practice personal and professional development plans.

Barbara Hawksley started her nursing career as a general nurse and then became a health visitor, before moving on to her present post as a Principal Lecturer in Community Nursing at Staffordshire University. Her experiences have given her a wide perspective of the range of possible treatment approaches and a belief in the importance of promoting self-help to the general public.

Gill Smith qualified as a radiographer. Over the past ten years she has branched out into researching musculoskeletal diseases and auditing various aspects of health at work in the NHS and other workplaces. Ruth and Gill have undertaken research that demonstrated the need for occupational health services for those working in primary care and the NHS workforce in general.

Chris Chambers has been a community physiotherapist for 20 years. One part of his duties has been to teach others about lifting and manual handling. Chris uses manipulation in his everyday clinical practice. More latterly he has developed an expertise in acupuncture, which he frequently uses in his NHS and private practice.

Acknowledgements

The development of this book and the integral educational programme has been funded as one of the Department of Health's *Back in Work* initiatives to 'promote good practice in back care management . . . that includes prevention, assessment, treatment and rehabilitation'.

The authors are grateful to those working in the NHS who have helped to pilot and critique this programme. In particular: community pharmacy advisor Jan Butterworth, community pharmacy tutor Carol Heydon and pharmacist Martyn Drew, GP Dr Gill Wakley and associate adviser in general practice Dr Mike Fisher, and practice managers Yvonne Bell and Gail Stanyer. Dr Steve Field, director of postgraduate general practice education at the West Midlands region, kindly accredited the programme and waived fees for GPs undertaking the pilot personal development plans. Dr Gill Wakley kindly scrutinised the manuscript for us.

Introduction to the book and the continuing professional development programme

The material in this book sets out how learning more about back pain and reviewing current practice can be incorporated into the personal development plans (PDPs) of GPs, pharmacists, nurses and practice managers. As part of the recent NHS changes, all health professionals and non-clinical staff should produce a PDP each year. A PDP will include details of identified learning needs, a timetabled learning action plan, evidence of progress and achievement – kept as a personal portfolio.

There is a dual focus on best practice in the clinical management of back pain and on improving the working environment for everybody – GP and pharmacist employers, staff, patients and customers. The book is relevant to you whether your working environment is a general medical practice, an independent pharmacy or one of a chain, a nursing home or patients' own homes. Practice teams should work together to direct their individual learning plans to form their practice personal or professional development plan (PPDP) that complements the business plan of the practice or pharmacy or that of their primary care group (PCG) or trust (PCT).[1]

This programme is focused on back pain because back pain is the largest single cause of ill health at work and sickness absence. 'Occupational health' aims to be proactive in promoting health and protecting the worker against occupationally acquired illness, rather than simply reacting to medical or environmental problems as they arise. 'Good occupational health practice . . . should lead, in the longer term, to positive outcomes for workers and businesses alike, in terms of a good quality of life inside and outside work, the social and material advantages of work, reduced sickness absence, higher productivity, a good, responsible image for individual businesses and greater national wealth creation.'[2]

There are two sides to occupational health:

- the effects of work and the workplace on health
- the effects of ill health on an individual's fitness for work.

You may decide to allocate 50% of the time you intend to spend drawing up, justifying and applying a PDP in any one year on best practice in back pain. That would leave space in your learning plan for other important topics, such as coronary heart disease, mental health or cancer – whatever is a priority for you, your post and your patient population.

Chapter 1 of the book describes how a clinical governance culture incorporates good clinical management and healthy/safe organisational or environmental working conditions.[3] You should be able to demonstrate that you are fit to practise as an individual clinician or manager (best practice in the management of back pain); and that your working environment is fit to practise from (a healthy and safe practice or pharmacy). This section will be relevant to all readers, whether you are a clinician, employer or manager, so that you understand more of the context within which you work and how your individual contribution fits into the whole picture of healthcare.

Chapter 2 describes why it is important to make learning about back pain a priority for your PDP or practice-team learning. Key facts about low back pain are given – how common and costly it is, how back pain arises, what to look for, what investigations to do and when. This chapter will be most relevant to GPs, nurses and pharmacists who provide clinical care. But the material has been written in a way that assumes little prior clinical knowledge so that it is relevant for practice managers who need to know more about back pain, about preventing back problems in their staff and about minimising hazards or problems in those already suffering.

Chapter 3 is devoted to the clinical management of low back pain, describing the evidence for best practice in the prevention and management of back pain: medication, physical therapies, mental therapies and other treatments that include conventional NHS and complementary treatments, and self-care. This will be relevant to GPs, pharmacists and nurses in their roles as health professionals caring for individual patients or customers. Anyone who suffers from back pain themselves will find the evidence for what works interesting, and that may give them ideas for what else they could try for themselves.

Chapter 4 describes what people in general or employees can do to look after their own backs. Employees are legally required to be aware of, and abide by, health and safety legislation. Knowing what to look for should help employees reduce back pain and likely hazards. These pages might be photocopied for individual members of staff in a GP practice or pharmacy, or patients and customers, to encourage self-care and enable them to review the health and safety of their own working environment.

Chapter 5 covers how GP and pharmacist employers or practice managers should adopt best practice in respect of health and safety at work in their practice or pharmacy. It shows practice managers how to develop a robust health and safety document for their practice. As the programme is focusing on back pain, the aspects considered include general health and safety, ergonomics and posture, manual handling, personal safety, reporting of accidents and injuries, and disability discrimination.

The whole programme builds up to the composing of a PDP or practice PPDP in Chapters 6 and 7. Interactive exercises throughout and at the end of each chapter give you, the reader, an opportunity to undertake an assessment of your learning needs, review your own performance or the safety of your workplace, and reflect on what improvements you could make. Simple risk assessments of the workplace, audits, challenges and other exercises encourage review and reflection.

You should transfer information from these needs assessment exercises to the relevant slots in the PDP if you are doing this programme as an individual, or the practice PPDP if you are working as a team. Adopt a wide-based approach to improving quality – think of how you are establishing a clinical governance culture in your own practice or pharmacy team in your timed action plans.

What should you do next?

Complete the baseline self-assessment of your knowledge and practice, given on pages xi–xiv. It will be good for you to look back to this assessment when you have completed your PDP or practice learning plan to realise the knowledge and skills you have gained, or changes you have made in the practice or pharmacy. Section A asks you about your current knowledge and practice in the clinical management of back pain. Section B asks you about your current knowledge and practice with respect to health and safety relevant to preventing back pain and problems in staff working in your practice or pharmacy.

Then study the template for a personal development plan on pages 107–110 or a practice personal and professional development plan on pages 133–136. You will be filling one of these in as you go along. Decide if you will be concentrating on the clinical management of back pain, or improving your working environment. It is unlikely you will have the time or inclination to do both – although you might, of course.

As you learn more about each topic, make changes as a result – to your workplace, or to the equipment in your practice which might be provoking back problems, or to the advice you give patients or customers, or the way you manage and investigate back pain or other back problems. Evaluate whether what you change makes a difference.

Baseline self-assessment of your knowledge and practice

Back pain matters: an educational programme to improve clinical management of back pain and/or health and safety at work

Let's get a snapshot of your current knowledge. Complete this before you start. Then you will be able to see how your learning improves your practice. If you are not sure of the answers, just tick the box that indicates that. Don't worry if you find you don't know very much – that's why you are learning about back pain now.

Complete either or both sections about clinical management of back pain or health and safety in your practice or pharmacy.

A Clinical management of back pain

1 When a patient presents with severe back pain do you advise exercise?

Usually   Sometimes   Rarely   Never   Not sure

2 Can you list five causes of back pain?

  i

  ii

  iii

  iv

  v

Not sure

3   What symptoms or history (e.g. cancer elsewhere) might indicate a serious condition is causing back pain rather than it being a simple muscular backache? Try to list at least five:

   i

   ii

   iii

   iv

   v

   Not sure

4   What do you know of the evidence for best practice in clinical management of back pain? List three key messages that direct your management:

   i

   ii

   iii

   Not sure

5   Have you undertaken an audit of any aspect of your clinical management of back pain in the last two years?

Referrals to others	Yes	No
Referrals for lumbar and/or sacral spine X-ray	Yes	No
Prescribed treatment	Yes	No

6   Do you refer patients with back pain to complementary or alternative therapists?

   Usually   Sometimes   Rarely   Never

   If you do, how much do you know about complementary or alternative therapy that is available locally? Do you know what alternative or complementary therapy is available, what the practitioners offer and what their qualifications are?

   Yes, good knowledge   Scant knowledge   No idea

Now complete the snapshop quiz (below) of your current knowledge or practice with health and safety relating to back pain

B Health and safety relating to back pain

1   Do you have a statement of your health and safety policy displayed in your premises for everyone to see?

Yes   No   Not sure

2   Have all your staff been instructed in manual handling?

Yes   No   Not sure

3   Has a risk assessment of your premises been carried out in the last year?

Yes   No   Not sure

3a If a risk assessment has been carried out, were any risks or hazards identified?

Yes   No   Not sure

3b What were the risks or hazards (list the three that were most important if there were many)?

i

ii

iii

Not sure

3c What changes were made as a result of identifying these risks or hazards?

i

ii

iii

Not sure

4 Do you have any trouble spots in your practice or pharmacy that might trigger back pain? Please tick any of those items listed below that are present in your workplace:

Trailing wires
Staff carry piles of papers or a load that is awkward or heavy for them
Staff sit with poor posture
Workstations uncomfortable – no chair with good support in front of every computer
Objects or piles of papers left lying on floor – in your office, staff room, back office
Temporary repairs to chairs or cupboards
Other (you add):

5 Have any of your staff or colleagues needed to take time off because of back pain during the last six months?

Yes   No   Not sure

(if so, how many days were lost? . . . .)

CHAPTER ONE

Clinical governance and the management of back pain

Clinical governance is inclusive – making quality everyone's business, whether a doctor or a nurse, a pharmacist or other independent contractor, manager, member of staff or a strategic planner. We need to know where we are now and where we want to get to if we are to drive up standards of healthcare.

Clinical governance is doing 'anything and everything required to maximise quality'.[3,4] Clinical governance should create a culture and working environment where people thrive and feel fulfilled by their work but where at the same time, underperformance is weeded out.

Components of clinical governance[3]

The components of clinical governance are not new. Bringing them together under the banner of clinical governance and introducing more explicit accountability for performance is a new style of working.

The following 14 themes are core components of professional and service development, which, taken together, form a comprehensive approach to providing high-quality healthcare services and clinical governance.[3] These are illustrated in the tree diagram in Figure 1.1. If you interweave these into your individual and workplace-based personal and professional development plans you will have met the requirements for clinical governance at the same time.[1,3]

1 Learning culture: in the practice or pharmacy.
2 Research and development culture: in the practice or pharmacy or throughout the health service.

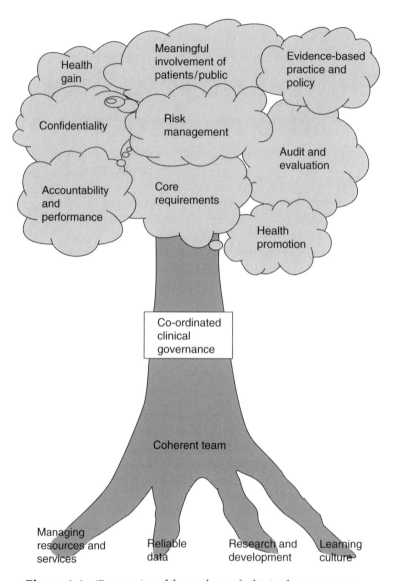

Figure 1.1: 'Routes' and branches of clinical governance.

3 Reliable and accurate data: in the practice, the pharmacy, the NHS as a seamless whole.
4 Well-managed resources and services: as individuals, as a practice, as a pharmacy, across the NHS and in conjunction with other organisations.
5 Coherent team: well-integrated teams within a practice or pharmacy, including attached staff.

6 Meaningful involvement of patients and the public: including users, carers and the general population.

7 Health gain: activities to improve the health of staff and patients in a practice, between practices, in a pharmacy.

8 Confidentiality: of information in consultations, in medical notes, between practitioners.

9 Evidence-based practice and policy: applying it in practice, in the pharmacy, in the district, across the NHS.

10 Accountability and performance: for standards, performance of individuals, the practice or pharmacy – to the public and those in authority.

11 Core requirements: good fit with skill-mix and whether individuals are competent to do their jobs, communication, workforce numbers, morale at practice or pharmacy level.

12 Health promotion: for patients, the public, your staff and colleagues – opportunistic and in general, targeting those with most needs.

13 Audit and evaluation: for instance of extent to which individuals and practice teams adhere to best practice in clinical management or human resources.

14 Risk management: for example competence in spotting 'red flags' (*see* Chapter 2), risk reduction of hazards in respect of back pain.

The challenges to delivering clinical governance

Delivering high-quality healthcare with guaranteed minimum standards of care for users at all times is a major challenge. At present, the quality of healthcare is patchy and variable. We are not very good at detecting underperformance and then taking the initiative and rectifying it at an early stage. The small number of clinicians who do underperform exert a disproportionately large effect on the public's confidence. Causes of underperformance in an individual might be a result of a lack of knowledge or skills, poor attitudes or ill health. A lack of management capability is nearly always an important contributory factor to inadequate clinical services.

We need to understand why variation exists and explore ways of reducing inequalities. Variation in the quality of healthcare provided is common – between different practices in the same locality, between staff of the same discipline working in the same practice or unit, between care given to some groups of the population rather than others. For example:

- the rates of referral to hospital may differ fourfold between one doctor and another for the same condition
- some general practices can refer directly to physiotherapists, while others have to refer to hospital first.

Clinical governance offers a co-ordinated approach to overcoming these areas of risk through the blend of clinical and organisational improvements to the quality of healthcare practice.

Learning culture: clinical governance component 1

Education and training programmes should be relevant to service needs, whether at organisational or individual levels. Continuing professional development (CPD) programmes need to meet both the learning needs of individual health professionals and the wider service development needs of the NHS. You should no longer opt for CPD activities according to what you *want* to do, but rather, what you *need* to do. Clinical governance underpins professional and service development.

---

individual personal development plans
will feed into a
**workplace- or practice-based personal and
professional development plan**
that will feed into
the organisation's business plan
all
underpinned by clinical governance[1]

So focusing on back pain would be a good topic for a practice PPDP with a mix of learning about the effective clinical management of back pain in a healthy and safe work environment.

Applying research and development in practice: clinical governance component 2

The conclusions of the many hundreds of research papers about back pain that are published in reputable journals each year are rarely applied in practice. This is because few health professionals or managers make time to read such journals systematically, and most are not therefore aware of the research findings. Neither do most practice or pharmacy teams have a system for reviewing important research papers and translating that review into practical action. The PCG/T might help by feeding important new evidence to its constituent practices or pharmacies, or indeed the general public, with suggestions or templates for making changes in practice, backed by resources to enable change to happen.

> Incorporating research-based evidence into everyday practice should promote policies on effective working, improve quality and expand the clinical governance culture.

Reliable and accurate data: clinical governance component 3

Clinicians, patients and administrators need reliable and accurate data to connect individuals or their healthcare records to other knowledge that is relevant to the care of the patient.

Set standards for a general practice (or in a pharmacy as appropriate) to:

- keep records in chronological order
- summarise medical records; within a specified time period for records of new patients
- review dates for checks on medication; with audit in place to monitor standards adhered to and plan for underperformance if necessary
- use computers for diagnostic recording
- record information from external sources – hospital, other organisations – relevant to individual patients or practice/pharmacy.

Keep good written records of policies and audits that relate to health and safety in the practice or pharmacy. An inspection at any time should show what risk assessments have been undertaken and when, the risk reductions that followed, the extent of staff training undertaken and the future programme of monitoring.

Well-managed resources and services: clinical governance component 4

The things you need to achieve best practice should be in the right place at the right time and working correctly every time.

Set standards in your workplace for:

- access to premises and availability of services for people with special needs such as those with disability from back pain
- provision of routine and urgent appointments
- access to and provision for referral for investigation or treatment
- proactive monitoring of chronic illness and disability
- alternatives to face-to-face consultations
- consultation length.

The six primary care services to which the public requires access are: information, advice, triage and treatment, continuity of care, personal care and other services.[5]

Systems should be designed to prevent and detect errors. So keep systems simple and sensible, and inform everyone how systems operate so that they are less likely to bypass the system or make errors. This certainly applies to health and safety matters where staff might be tempted to cut corners and take risks, or to follow-up of patients' clinical management. *See* Appendix 1 for extracts from relevant legislation.

Coherent team work: clinical governance component 5

Teams produce better patient care than single practitioners operating in a fragmented way. Effective teams make the most of the different contributions of individual clinical disciplines in delivering patient care. The characteristics of effective teams are:

- shared ownership of a common purpose
- clear goals for the contributions each discipline makes
- open communication between team members
- opportunities for team members to enhance their skills.

A team approach helps different team members adopt an evidence-based approach to patient care – by having to justify their approach to the rest of the team.[6] Back pain is a good example of the need for teamwork to achieve the best results for individual patients, where primary care team members include: the GP and practice nurse, physiotherapist, non-clinical staff and community pharmacist.

Meaningful involvement of patients and the public: clinical governance component 6

People use terms like 'user' or 'consumer' or 'customer' to describe who we should be involving in giving us feedback about the quality or type of healthcare we offer, or in planning future services. Patients or carers, non-users of services, the local community, a particular subgroup of the population or the general public will all have useful feedback and views; for example, on the safety of your own practice or pharmacy premises, or your systems for informing people about the results of investigations or queries.

If user involvement and public participation is done well it should result in:

- reductions in health inequalities
- better outcomes of individual care
- better health for the population
- better quality and more locally responsive services
- greater ownership of health services
- a better understanding of why and how local services need to be changed and developed.

A meaningful public consultation involves the exchange of information between the healthcare providers and the general public. A representative opinion is obtained that feeds into the local decision-making process of healthcare services or whoever is sponsoring the consultation. For example, you might want to consult the public and health professionals about the availability of complementary therapies in the NHS.

You may have to trade off a relatively cheaper method of consultation that engages with fewer people or with a less representative section of the population subgroup. If you do, you will need to understand what biases are arising and make allowances for them when you interpret the results of the consultation.[7]

Health gain: clinical governance component 7

The two general approaches to improving health are the 'population' approach, focusing on measures to improve health through the community, and the 'high-risk' approach, focusing on vulnerable individuals who are at high risk of the condition or hazard.

The two approaches are not mutually exclusive and often need to be combined with legislation and community action. Health goals include:

- a good quality of life
- avoiding premature death
- equal opportunities for health.

Modifiable risk factors for reducing the likelihood of back pain at work include:

- poor posture, e.g. sitting or standing
- poorly designed office furniture, e.g. a workstation where the chair is not at the right height for the reception counter or computer
- presence of physical hazards in the workplace, e.g. trailing wires
- obesity
- lack of exercise
- staff untrained in manual handling.

Confidentiality: clinical governance component 8

Confidentiality is a component of clinical governance that is often overlooked. Experienced health professionals and managers may assume that junior or new staff know all about confidentiality whereas, of course, they may not. There are many tricky situations in a practice or pharmacy where one person asks for information about another's medical condition – test results or a progress report – where it is not clear-cut as to whether this information should be supplied or withheld, or even if the person asked should acknowledge that the person enquired about is under their care.

The Caldicott committee report described principles of good practice to safeguard confidentiality when information is being used for non-clinical purposes[8]:

- justify the purpose
- do not use patient-identifiable information unless it is absolutely necessary
- use the minimum necessary patient-identifiable information
- access to patient-identifiable information should be on a strict need-to-know basis
- everyone with access to patient-identifiable information should be aware of his or her responsibilities.

Evidence-based culture – policy and practice: clinical governance component 9

The key features of whether or not local guidelines worked in one initiative[9] were that:

- there was multidisciplinary involvement in drawing them up
- a well-described systematic review of the literature underpinned the guidelines with graded recommendations for best practice linked to the evidence
- ownership was nurtured at a national and local level
- a local implementation plan ensured that all the practicalities (time, staff, education and training, resources) were foreseen and met, stakeholders were supported and predictors of sustainability addressed – guideline usability, individualising guidelines to practitioners and patients.

A study of 30 general practices in the Netherlands explored the extent to which GPs adhered to guidelines for the management of low back pain.[10] The study found that older patients were less likely to be examined, despite the increasing probability of finding serious pathology with increasing age. About three-quarters of GPs gave the recommended advice to remain active despite the pain, at initial and follow-up consultations.

Accountability and performance: clinical governance component 10

Health professionals may not always realise that they are accountable to others from outside their own professions, especially those who are self-employed, such as GPs and pharmacists. But in fact they are accountable to:

- the general public, who are entitled to expect high standards of healthcare
- the profession – to maintain standards of knowledge and skills of the profession as a whole
- the government – and employer – who expect high standards of healthcare from the workforce.

Health professionals who believe that they are not accountable to others may be reluctant to collect the evidence to demonstrate that they are fit to practise, and that their working environment is fit to practise from. They may be reluctant to co-operate with central NHS requirements such as working to the National Service Frameworks.

Identify and rectify underperformance at an early stage by:

- regular appraisals (at least annually) linked into clinical governance and PDPs. Appraisal may be carried out through regular meetings between manager and staff member, or doctor/pharmacist with an external or internal appraiser with support for the benefit of the member of staff being appraised
- detecting those who have significant health problems and referring them for help
- systematic audit that detects individuals' performance as opposed to the overall performance of the practice team
- an open learning culture where team members are discouraged from covering up colleagues' inadequacies so that problems can be resolved at an early stage.

Clinicians may see the performance assessment framework as a management tool that is not particularly relevant to their clinical practice. But it does reinforce a clinical governance culture whereby good clinical and organisational management have a symbiotic relationship.

> The NHS performance assessment framework has six components, which include: health improvement, fair access, efficiency, effective delivery of appropriate care, user/carer experience and health outcomes.

Health promotion:
clinical governance component 11

People may underestimate relative risks as applied to themselves and their own behaviour – for example, many smokers accept the relationship between smoking tobacco and disease, but do not believe that they are personally at risk. People usually have a reasonable idea of the *relative risks* of various activities and behaviours, although their personal estimates of the *magnitude* of risks tend to be biased – small probabilities are often overestimated and high probabilities are often underestimated.

> Some published research has suggested an association between cigarette smoking and the prevalence and severity of back pain. However, a systematic review of 41 journal articles concluded that smoking should be considered as a weak risk indicator and not a cause of low back pain.[11]

Obesity is associated with chronic or recurrent low back pain, especially in women; it is thought to play a part in the chronicity of simple low back pain rather than be an actual cause of the back pain arising.[12]

Audit and evaluation: clinical governance component 12

Audit will probably be the method you think of first for determining what your needs are – as a clinician or as a practice. You might look at the extent to which you are adhering to practice or pharmacy protocols – for instance whether you are consistently advising those with back pain to remain active or comparing other aspects of clinical care with best practice guidelines. Or you might audit the extent to which you comply with health and safety legislation.

> An audit of GP referrals for lumbar spine X-rays in Coventry achieved a 61% reduction in lumbar spine X-ray requests and an increased proportion of X-rays with positive results one year after the initial audit and an educational meeting to discuss radiology guidelines.[13]

Analysis of critical incidents should focus on organisational factors and the performance of particular individuals. For example, if a member of staff is off sick with back pain after an incident at work, a risk assessment and analysis of the workplace might reveal many areas where changes might be made to reduce potential hazards and a recurrence of the incident. Or if a patient taking non-steroidal anti-inflammatory drugs (NSAIDs) for back pain has a haematemesis, the treating GP or associated pharmacist might review their management of that individual to see if their usual approach conforms with best practice as recommended in national guidelines.

Core requirements: clinical governance component 13

You cannot deliver clinical governance without well-trained and competent staff, the right skill-mix of staff, a safe and comfortable working environment, and cost-effective care. Following published referral guidelines may increase healthcare costs, which should be justifiable as cost-effective care when all direct and indirect costs are taken into account.

Your healthcare team can do much under the umbrella of clinical governance to respond to the government challenges to improve:

- partnership: working together across the NHS to ensure the best possible care
- performance: acting to review and deliver higher standards of healthcare
- the professions and wider workforce: breaking down barriers between different disciplines, for instance through multidisciplinary team-work between GPs and nurses with pharmacists
- patient care: access, convenient services, empowerment to take full part in decision making about their own medical care and in planning and providing health services in general
- prevention: promoting healthy living across all sections of society and tackling variations in care.

Risk management: clinical governance component 14

Risk management in general practice or the pharmacy mainly centres on assessing probabilities that potential or actual hazards will give rise to harm – how bad is the risk, how likely is the risk, when will the risk happen if ever and how certain are you of estimates about the risks? This applies just as much, whether the risk is an environmental or organisational risk in the practice, or a clinical risk.

Good practice means understanding and managing risk – both clinical and organisational aspects. Undertaking audit more system-atically will reduce the risks of omission – in detection and clinical management. The common areas of risk in providing healthcare services are thought to be[14]:

- out-of-date clinical practice
- lack of continuity of care
- poor communication
- mistakes in patient care
- patient complaints
- financial risk – insufficient resources
- reputation
- staff morale.

Communicating and managing risks with individual patients is very much about finding ways to explain risks and elicit people's values and preferences so that all these dimensions can be incorporated into the decisions they make for themselves to take risks or to choose between alternatives that involve different risks and benefits. A well-functioning system through which patients can make complaints and receive feedback on the outcome should allow the practice or unit to reduce risks of a recurrence.

Reflection exercises

Exercise 1. Reviewing and planning your clinical management of back pain

Think how you might integrate the 14 components of clinical governance into your PDP. Examples are given for each component listed below. Have a go at completing this yourself from your own perspective.

- *Establishing a learning culture*: e.g. informal discussion session about back-pain guidelines between GPs, nurses and community pharmacist.
- *Managing resources and services*: e.g. mapping of practitioners to whom patients/customers can be referred; informing PCG/T of shortfalls in numbers of therapists.
- *Establishing a research and development culture*: e.g. sharing findings in key research papers on best practice in back pain with colleagues.
- *Reliable and accurate data*: e.g. keep electronic records in consistent way (self and team) so that any audit exercises can be repeated next year and results compared.
- *Evidence-based practice and policy*: e.g. draw up or contribute to an evidence-based protocol on back pain, including promotion of self-care, medication, clinical management.
- *Confidentiality*: e.g. giving results or advice at the reception desk or counter.
- *Health gain*: e.g. obtain or write literature promoting exercise – local walks, health messages.
- *Coherent team*: e.g. communicating new systems to rest of team.
- *Audit and evaluation*: e.g. undertaking audit and acting on findings to improve quality.

- *Meaningful involvement of patients and the public*: e.g. listening to and acting on patients' comments about your clinical care or service.
- *Health promotion*: e.g. promoting best practice in self-care: exercise and good posture.
- *Risk management*: e.g. establishing systems and procedures to identify, analyse and control any or all of the risks in clinical management, such as repeat prescribing, overinvestigation.
- *Accountability and performance*: e.g. keeping good records to demonstrate best practice.
- *Core requirements*: e.g. agreeing roles and responsibilities in a team, such as when nurses and physiotherapists should refer patients to GPs, training counter assistants to give reliable advice.

Exercise 2. Reviewing and planning health and safety in your practice or pharmacy

Think how you might integrate the 14 components of clinical governance into your PDP or practice learning plan. Examples are given for each component listed below. Have a go at completing this from your perspective.

- *Establishing a learning culture*: e.g. session updating staff at multidisciplinary meeting.
- *Managing resources and services*: e.g. investing in new equipment or workstations.
- *Establishing a research and development culture*: e.g. find out what hazards patients or customers have noted in your practice or pharmacy.
- *Reliable and accurate data*: e.g. record risk assessment in clear, consistent way so that the exercise can be repeated next year and results compared.
- *Evidence-based practice and policy*: e.g. formulate a protocol for minimising back-pain problems among your staff based on policies for health and safety or manual handling.
- *Confidentiality*: e.g. take care with records of health and wellbeing of your staff.
- *Health gain*: e.g. from reducing staff exposure to hazards and risks.
- *Coherent team*: e.g. communicating new systems and procedures well.
- *Audit and evaluation*: e.g. undertaking regular audits and acting on findings.

- *Meaningful involvement of patients and the public*: e.g. acting on patients' comments.
- *Health promotion*: e.g. promoting best practice in manual handling to staff.
- *Risk management*: e.g. establishing systems and procedures to identify, analyse and control any or all of the risks found after risk assessment of the workplace.
- *Accountability and performance*: e.g. keeping good records to demonstrate that the working environment is safe.
- *Core requirements*: e.g. agreeing roles and responsibilities in team for the various health and safety policies and tasks.

Now that you have completed one or more of the interactive reflection exercises in this chapter, transfer the information from this needs assessment to the empty template of the PDP on pages 107–110 if you are working on your own learning plan; or to the practice PPDP on pages 133–136 if you are working on a practice-team learning plan. The conclusions made at the end of each exercise will feature in the action plan. Don't forget to keep evidence of your learning in your personal portfolio.

CHAPTER TWO

Key facts about back pain and best practice in clinical management

Back pain is common and costly

Back pain is a very common condition. Over 70% of people in developed countries experience low back pain at some time in their lives.[15] Overall, about 16.5 million people in the UK suffer from back pain in any one year. Most people can deal with their back pain themselves most of the time.[16] In a typical year, about three to seven million back pain sufferers are thought to consult a GP about their back pain at least once, 1.6 million people attend hospital-based outpatients, about 100 000 are admitted to hospital and 24 000 have surgery for back pain. About 7% of the adult population in the UK present to their GP with back pain in any one year.[16]

Two in every five adults in the UK report suffering from back pain lasting more than one day in the previous 12 months. Of the people who reported back pain in one study, one-sixth said they were in pain throughout the year, and a third described back pain as having restricted their activities in the previous month.[17]

Low back pain is usually self-limiting. Ninety percent of people with low back pain recover within six weeks, but 2–7% of people develop chronic pain. Once a person has been off work with back pain for six months, they have about a 50% chance of getting back to work.[15]

The estimated annual cost to the NHS of back pain in a GP practice of 10 000 patients was approximately £88 000 in 1993.[16] This was made up of:

- 440 outpatient clinic visits   £13 000
- 150 inpatient days   £20 000
- prescribed drugs   £8000
- 2180 GP consultations   £23 700
- 1270 physical therapy sessions   £11 000
- 90 A and E attendances   £3000
- X-rays   £8000

During the decade to 1993, outpatient attendances in Britain rose fivefold, and the number of days' incapacity from back disorders for which social security benefits were paid more than doubled.[18] Researchers investigating this trend found that although more people reported having back pain over a ten-year period, there was no corresponding rise in the numbers of people who reported being unable to put on hosiery (socks, stockings or tights), which was taken as a proxy indicator of disabling back pain or problems. They concluded that the increase in reported back pain did not reflect an associated greater incidence of severe back disease.

Back pain affects people in all types of workplaces. The highest incidence is in the retail, food, construction, water and health service sectors, as well as in mining and agriculture.

It is estimated that back pain accounts for about 100 million lost working days per year in the UK and around £500 million in health and welfare costs.[19]

Who suffers from back pain?

Low back pain is most common in people aged 35 to 55 years old. About a third of people in professional and skilled non-manual occupations report back pain; less than the 50% or so of those in manual and unskilled jobs who experience back pain.

Back pain was given as the reason for taking time off work in the previous month by one in 20 of the back-pain sufferers in one survey,[17] and for one in six was the reason why they said they were not in employment. About half of those who stay off work with back pain return to work after a few days.

Defining back pain

The symptoms of backache or back pain depend on what the cause is, whether the pain arises from the spine or muscles around the spine, or whether a nerve is trapped at its root so that pain radiates down the nerve to the leg and on to the foot.

Low back pain is the term given to a mix of symptoms, including pain felt in the small of the back. Back pain of up to six weeks' duration is classified arbitrarily as 'acute'. It is common for someone who suffers from acute back pain to experience recurrences of back pain.[20]

> Low back pain is 'pain, muscle tension, or stiffness localised below the costal margin and above the inferior gluteal folds, with or without leg pain (sciatica)'.[20]

Non-specific low back pain is 'low back pain not attributed to recognisable pathology such as infection, tumour, osteoporosis, rheumatoid arthritis, fracture or inflammation'.[20]

'Simple backache' describes back pain with a mechanical origin. That is, the pain originates from the bony structure of the spine or the muscles attached to it. Symptoms vary with different physical activities and time of day. Simple backache can be very painful; the pain may spread in a general way down to one or both hips, thighs and legs. The difference between simple backache and other types of back pain is that the lumbar or sciatic nerve roots or the spinal cord are not compressed.

> **Features of simple backache**
> - Onset is usually between the ages of 20 and 55 years old
> - Pain is in the lumbosacral region, buttocks and thighs
> - Pain is mechanical in nature: varies with physical activity and over time
> - Person is well
> - Outlook is good: 90% recover from an acute attack in six weeks

Chronic back pain is variably defined as back pain that persists for longer than seven to 12 weeks or 'pain that lasts beyond the expected period of healing'.[21] Data about the epidemiology of chronic low back pain is uncertain. Five to 10% of the population in the UK continue to have some degree of back pain over long periods of their lives. Three to 4% of the population aged 16 to 44 and 5–7% of those aged 45 to 64 report back problems as a 'chronic sickness'.[15] Chronic back pain is sometimes used as a diagnosis of convenience by people who are actually disabled for socio-economic, work-related or psychological reasons.[21]

Nerve root pain

Nerve root pain is usually caused by a disc prolapse, spinal stenosis or scarring from previous surgery, which is causing compression of a nerve. Less than 5% of sufferers have sciatica, which is due to the sciatic nerve root being compressed and causing the pain. The pain from the compressed nerve root is localised to a particular site down one leg, which corresponds with the skin-ending of that strand of the nerve. Sciatic pain commonly radiates down one leg to the foot or toes, following the path of the left or right branch of the sciatic nerve from the lumbar and sacral spine to the foot on the same side of the body. Numbness and pins and needles are often associated with the distribution of the pain. Sometimes sensation is lost around the same area, or the muscle is weaker or the reflex of the muscle brisker.

Features of nerve root pain

- One-sided leg pain may be worse than back pain
- Pain usually radiates down to foot or toes
- Numbness and tingling in same path as leg/foot pain
- Signs that nerve root is irritated or compressed; raising leg with knee straight reproduces the leg pain
- Changes in muscle power, sensation and reflexes along pathway of nerve
- Reasonable outlook: 50% recover from an acute attack within six weeks

---

Causes of back pain

Most backache is simply pain arising from the spine or muscles around the spine. Pain is non-specific in about 85% of those presenting to primary care; about 4% have compression fractures, 1–3% have a prolapsed intervertebral disc and about 1% have a neoplasm.[20]

Poor posture

Sitting can cause the pelvis to rotate backwards causing the lumbar spine to bend, compressing the intervertebral discs and cartilage. Raising your arms in front of your body (for instance typing on a keyboard) or lifting objects while sitting increases this pressure even more. The damage may be compounded if the muscles around the spine holding the person in position become tired.

Bad lifting techniques

Poor lifting techniques can trigger damage and thus low back pain; a bent-back lift may produce twice as much force on the back compared to a bent-knee lift. The force on the intervertebral discs is increased still further by twisting at the same time. Lifting a heavy load increases the downwards stress on the spine, and the total stress is calculated by multiplying it by the distance A (the weight) to B (your spine). B is the point on the spine where most bending is taking place, i.e. the lumbar spine. If you make A–B longer, by bending over, the magnitude of the load increases dramatically. Acute back pain may be triggered by one single incident, such as lifting a heavy load, or repeated minor events, such as sitting hunched over a keyboard.

Being overweight

Being overweight or obese will pull the spine into an unnatural position which is more susceptible to wear and tear and may perpetuate back pain.

Arthritis or wear and tear or spondylitis

Sometimes the disc becomes narrower and the facet joints swell, so that movements become stiff and painful. Occasionally there is extra growth around the edges of the bone so that the nerve has a smaller space to pass through and may press on the bone. Treatment should be aimed at keeping as much movement as possible, especially that which increases the backwards curve of the lumbar spine.

Ankylosing spondylitis

This is an inflammatory condition that usually occurs in young men. Key symptoms are stiffness of the joints early in the morning, which is relieved by exercise or anti-inflammatory drugs. Other joints may be affected elsewhere.

Features of an inflammatory disorder

- Gradual onset of disorder
- Spinal stiffness worse in the morning
- Spine movements limited in all directions
- Other joints of the body involved – painful and stiff
- Skin rashes common, e.g. psoriasis
- Inflammation of the eye(s) (iritis) common
- Discharge from urethra typical, e.g. Reiters syndrome
- Colitis – inflamed colon causing diarrhoea
- Family history of the disorder

Slipped or prolapsed disc

This can be caused by poor posture, the result of a jarring accident or lifting something incorrectly. The jelly-like centre of the intervertebral disc can be forced through the outer rings of the disc because of excess vertical pressure on the spine. Typically, more pressure is put on the front of the disc so that the jelly is pushed backwards, but sometimes sideways slippage of the jelly can also occur. This can happen when sitting or standing for long periods with the lumbar spine flattened, instead of keeping the correct curve; alternatively, lifting a weight by bending forwards can put a similar strain on the front of the disc. The 'slipped' disc then presses on the nerve, giving pain. Pain or pins and needles may be felt along the path of the nerve, which could be in the buttock, thigh or foot.

Osteoporosis

Osteoporosis causes bone pain, especially in the spine, because the bones become thinner and may partly or fully collapse; this may give additional pain from the resulting curve or change in structure that compresses the nerve roots. It usually occurs in elderly people or in younger people who have other reasons for it, such as taking steroid drugs. Pain may come on suddenly after some minor knock or after bending over; the bones are so thin that such minor injury can cause a vertebra to collapse. The resulting pain is severe and lasts six to eight weeks before it starts to improve.

Other causes

There are other causes of back pain such as damage to the spine from a road accident or serious fall. Some people are born with a physical abnormality, such as an extra vertebra or one that develops unevenly giving an unusual curve to the spine. Bony pain may occur from spread from cancers. Pain from other organs in the body can radiate to the spine from the kidneys, ovaries, uterus or other abdominal organs.

Spinal tumours or infection, inflammatory diseases such as ankylosing spondylitis, structural deformities of the spine and generalised neurological disorders produce back pain, which is often constant and steadily worsens. This kind of pain is not related to physical activity and, as the conditions do not usually compress nerve roots, does not have the same pattern of pain as when a nerve root is compromised.

What to look for

History

A description of when the back pain started, the sites of pain, if it radiates down the legs, occupation, previous problems, medication, general health and lifestyle, or a recent injury all give clues to the cause, type of back pain and whether a person needs urgent investigation or simple treatment. Family history may be relevant if there is any particular joint problem common in the immediate family. There are some well-recognised 'red flags' that could indicate to a doctor or therapist that the back pain is a symptom of a serious condition (see box below).

'Red flags' indicating possible serious spinal pathology[22,23]

- significant injury, such as from a road traffic accident or fall from a height
- cancer elsewhere
- presenting with severe back pain for the first time under age 20 or over age 55 years
- generally unwell, weight loss
- being on steroid drugs or abusing drugs
- difficulty urinating
- thoracic pain
- widespread neurological signs and symptoms
- constant progressive non-mechanical pain
- structural deformity

The person's psychological state could affect how quickly he or she gets better and whether the back pain recurs. 'Yellow flags' indicate negative attitudes and beliefs and behaviours on the part of the person with back pain that may predict poor outcomes (see box below).

'Yellow flags' indicating psychosocial risk factors for back pain[22,23]

- a belief that back pain is harmful or potentially severely disabling
- avoiding movement because of fear of triggering the back pain
- reduced activity levels
- tendency to low mood
- withdrawal from social interaction
- opting for a passive treatment rather than actively participating in the treatment

---

In one study of two general practices, disabling low back pain was associated with: high levels of psychosocial distress, poor self-rated health, low levels of physical activity, dissatisfaction with employment, widespread pain and restriction in spinal mobility.[24]

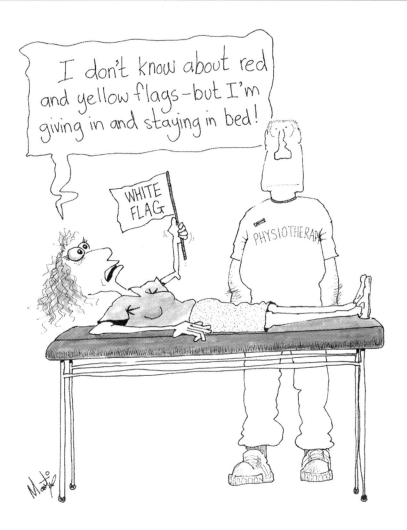

Examination[25]

The extent of the examination will vary depending on how concerned GPs or physiotherapists are about the histories patients give and whether or not they suspect a serious problem. Just looking at a patient's back should give more information about what could be wrong: look at the way the patient walks, whether or not the pelvis tilts forwards, if the shoulders are level with each other, and the curve of the spine when standing straight up. Raising each of the legs with the knees kept straight may be restricted, or that movement may reproduce the pain, or there may be significant degrees of muscle weakness. The spine may be pulled out of the contours of its usual curving structure by muscles around the spine contracting in response to the pain or cause. Physical examination includes: how the spine moves when the person flexes his or her trunk forwards with knees straight, or extends his or her back backwards or sideways or rotates it; and tests of sensation to look for other signs of nerve damage down the legs or around the buttocks and genital area. Signs of other conditions, such as other swollen or painful joints or skin rashes, may indicate a more general cause for the back pain from outside the spine, such as ankylosing spondylitis or other inflammatory disorders.

Investigations[25]

Blood tests

These would not be done routinely for simple back pain. If pain persists or a cause outside the spine is suspected, blood tests might detect or eliminate other conditions, such as cancers or various forms of arthritis. A raised erythrocyte sedimentation rate or plasma viscosity, a raised white cell count, raised alkaline or acid phosphates and a monoclonal band on electrophoresis of plasma all indicate serious disease.

X-rays

Acute back pain is usually due to conditions that cannot be diagnosed on a straight X-ray (except osteoporotic collapse). Routine X-rays are not recommended for investigating an acute episode of low back pain lasting less than six weeks unless there are unusual signs that alert the doctor or therapist to the possibility of a serious disease. Three standard X-ray views of the lumbar spine involve 120 to 150 times the radiation dose of a chest X-ray and should not be undertaken lightly; an estimated 19 deaths may arise from the 700 000 people in the UK who have lumbar spine radiographs each year.[22, 26]

Straight X-rays of the thoracic, lumbar or sacral spine are useful if a fracture, tumour, infection or osteoporosis is suspected. There is no need for a back to be X-rayed before a therapist undertakes manipulation. X-rays are not a good guide to how severe arthritis is; plenty of people whose spine X-rays show wear and tear changes have few or no symptoms, just as there are people who complain of a great deal of back pain and are believed to have osteoarthritis, who have normal-looking X-rays. People can have serious conditions such as early cancer affecting their bones and the X-rays look normal, because it takes time for diseases such as cancer or infection to destroy the bone sufficiently for this to show up on an X-ray.

Guidelines on appropriate use of radiology in relation to back pain[22]

1 Plain X-rays are not recommended for routine evaluation of patients with acute low back problems of less than six weeks duration unless a 'red flag' is noted on clinical examination.
2 Plain X-rays of the lumbar spine are recommended for ruling out fractures in patients with acute back problems when any of the following 'red flags' are present: recent significant trauma (any age), recent mild trauma (patient over age 50), prolonged steroid use, osteoporosis, patient over 70 years old.
3 Plain X-rays in combination with full blood count and erythrocyte sedimentation rate may be useful for ruling out tumour or infection in patients with acute low back problems when any of the following 'red flags' are present: prior cancer or recent infection, fever over 37.8°C (100°F), intravenous drug abuse, low back pain worse with rest, unexplained weight loss, prolonged steroid use.
4 The routine use of oblique views on plain lumbar X-rays is not recommended because of the increased exposure to radiation.

Isotope bone scans

These are recommended when a spinal tumour, infection or a previously undetected fracture is suspected from the medical history or physical examination and has been corroborated by blood tests or X-ray findings.

Magnetic resonance imaging scanning

A magnetic resonance imaging (MRI) scan is a highly specialised test and is only justified when there are clinical indications of a sinister problem with the spine, or before surgery is carried out. An MRI scan is generally preferred to computerised tomography (CT) as it gives a wider field of view and avoids X-irradiation. Myelography may be useful for delineating a tumour prior to operation.

When to refer to a specialist

Surgery is rarely to be recommended and should only be considered where conservative treatment has failed. The main role of spinal surgery is for the treatment of nerve root problems that are not getting better or where the compression is at such a level and is so great that the patient has difficulty urinating, retaining their faeces, and has widespread loss of sensation and muscle tone around the genital area and legs (the 'cauda equina' syndrome).

> One study of all new outpatient attendances for low back pain during one month in two hospitals showed how disorganised GP referrals were. Patients with low back pain accounted for 15–20% of all new outpatient attendances. The patients were seen in at least ten specialties and two-fifths of them had been seen previously with the same symptom in another department. The authors of the study called for a more coherent referral policy.[27]

In England, the number of surgical operations on the spine increased from 11 000 in 1982 to 17 223 in 1989–90.[15]

Consider making a surgical referral for:

- nerve root pain – if this is not resolving within four weeks, specialist referral may be appropriate; manipulation can be used where progressive neurological deficit is ruled out. Non-responding or deteriorating cases should be referred for orthopaedic or neurosurgical opinion as appropriate
- possible serious spinal pathology – if 'red flags' suggest possible serious pathology, prompt investigations should exclude this, or lead to referral to a specialist within four weeks
- cauda equina syndrome – this is a medical emergency requiring immediate referral, if necessary through an accident and emergency department.

Other therapists

People with back pain may choose to pay for private treatment with a physiotherapist, osteopath or chiropractor as the first-line practitioner. Referral for treatment on the NHS by a GP will be influenced by availability, personal preferences, knowledge of local practitioners and the evidence base.

See later sections for the evidence on types and timing of physical therapies.

Outcomes of treatment

Simple backache in reasonably well 20- to 55-year-olds, which is 'mechanical' in nature, varying with physical activity and time of day, has a good outlook, with at least 90% recovering from an acute episode within six weeks. Back pain due to a nerve root being compressed in the spine does not have such a good outlook, with only 50% recovering from the acute episode within six weeks.[15]

Key information points for people with simple backache

- There is nothing to worry about, backache is very common
- Not a sign of any serious damage or disease
- Full recovery in days or weeks – but may vary
- No permanent weakness. Recurrence is possible – but this does not mean a reinjury has occurred
- Activity is helpful, too much rest is not. Hurting does not mean harm

---

Most cases of severe back pain with severe limitation of activity improve considerably in a few days, or at most a few weeks; but milder symptoms may persist for longer, often for a few months.

Early rehabilitation of patients with low back pain can prevent the development of chronic pain.

Most back-pain sufferers will have some recurrences of back pain from time to time. Recurrences are to be expected and do not mean that they have re-injured their back or that their condition is getting worse. The checklist in the box overleaf gives the risk factors for chronic back pain. There is a great deal individuals can do to improve their physical health and general wellbeing to reduce the chances of back pain recurring. Advise people to stop smoking, increase their fitness, build up their muscles, find ways of improving general satisfaction with life and work, and control the stresses in their life. People who have a positive attitude to life and do not unduly dwell upon their ill health or disabilities have more chance of minimising the effects of back pain and other illnesses. Back pain sufferers who return to their normal activities feel healthier, use fewer pain killers and are less distressed by their back pain, compared to those who limit their daily activities.

Risk factors for chronic back pain[22]

- Previous history of low back pain
- Significant time lost from work due to low back pain in previous 12 months
- Radiating leg pain
- Reduced straight leg raising
- Signs of nerve root involvement
- Reduced muscle strength and endurance of trunk
- Poor physical fitness
- Self-rated health is poor
- Heavy smoking
- Psychological distress and depressive symptoms
- Disproportionate illness behaviour
- Low job satisfaction
- Personal problems: alcohol, marital and financial
- Adversarial medico-legal proceedings

Reflection exercises

Exercise 3 (for GPs, pharmacists or community nurses). Is learning more about low back pain a priority for you or your practice team? Is it a district or national priority?

State why you have given the answer you have:

Justify why you should include learning about low back pain in your PDP. Choose one or several of the activities listed below to determine topics and areas about which you need to learn more:

- analyse a recent significant event (for example, a patient with back pain has not been investigated for six months when metastatic disease is eventually found)
- undertake a SWOT analysis of your current knowledge and skills in the clinical management of back pain, describing strengths, weaknesses, opportunities and threats
- sit in with another professional at work – hospital consultant, GP, pharmacist, physiotherapist – to find out more about what you don't know you don't know
- undertake an audit of your current practice and compare with national guidelines (for example, advice you give about exercise)
- read a few key articles from the references or reading list given at the end of the book. Make notes about any new information you learn and plan how to apply that in your practice.

Exercise 4 (for GPs)

Photocopy the pages of this exercise – one for each patient reviewed.

(i) Undertake an audit of patients who have been referred for X-ray investigations and compare with national guidelines (*see* page 27)

Review the notes of 20 consecutive patients with back pain who present to you in the practice and are consulting you at a follow-up appointment about their back pain (although this may not be their only reason for the consultation). You will need to have seen the patient at least once before, irrespective of whether the patient has consulted other GPs in your practice too. Review for how many you (or a colleague) ordered a lumbar or lumbar-sacral spine X-ray. Look at the reasons why an X-ray was arranged and how those reasons compare with the guidelines described on page 27.

If less than five of your cohort of 20 consecutive patients were referred for a lumbar or lumbar-sacral spine X-ray, collect and review the next five X-ray reports landing on your desk too.

For each patient:

1 Were any 'red flag' symptoms present to justify the X-ray?   Yes/No
2 How long had the back pain been present?
3 What was the reason for investigation?

4 Was there any change of management as a result of the X-ray findings?

Conclude: are you referring patients for X-ray investigations in accordance with recommended best practice?[26] Have you any need to learn more about appropriate X-ray investigation? Will it be worthwhile repeating your audit in a year's time?

(ii) Undertake an audit of patients who have been referred to a hospital consultant, physiotherapist, chiropractor or osteopath

Use the notes of the 20 consecutive patients with back pain being followed up who you reviewed in Exercise 4(i) above. Include all NHS and private referrals, and do not distinguish between referrals to a community therapist who is sited in your practice and one working in another primary care site or a hospital base.

For each patient:

1 Was the patient referred to an orthopaedic or other hospital specialist? Yes/No

If yes, why was this?

- Nerve root pain not resolving
- Possible serious spinal pathology
- Cauda equina syndrome
- Other (please state):

2 What treatment did the patient receive?

Does this comply with recommendations for best practice?[22,23]

If not, do you know why not?

3 Was the patient referred for physiotherapy/osteopathy/chiropractic?
Yes/No

If 'yes', what was the reason for the referral?

• Patient's pain required further intervention   Yes/No
• Patient was unlikely to return to normal activities
within six weeks?   Yes/No
• Patient was unlikely to return to work within six weeks? Yes/No
• Second opinion as to the cause of back pain required   Yes/No
• Other reason:

Conclude: are you referring patients to hospital specialists or NHS/ private therapists in accordance with recommended best practice?[22,23] Do you need to learn more about making appropriate referrals – would you benefit from reviewing your practice protocol with those to whom you do or can refer?

Now that you have completed one or more of the interactive reflection exercises in this chapter, transfer the information from this needs assessment to the empty template of the PDP on pages 107–110 if you are working on your own learning plan, or to the PPDP on pages 133–136 if you are working on a practice-team learning plan. The conclusions made at the end of each exercise will feature in the action plan. Don't forget to keep evidence of your learning in your personal portfolio.

CHAPTER THREE

The range of physical, mental and oral treatments and the evidence where it is known

There is a growing body of evidence about which treatments work to reduce back pain and improve mobility. More research has been carried out to study the conventional types of NHS treatments than alternative or complementary therapies. Reports of research and reviews of studies can be misleading. Some researchers are selective in reporting the results of their studies – academic journals are more likely to publish results of successful treatments rather than studies that show no benefits.

There are four physical approaches to helping back pain:

- controlling the symptoms of pain and stiffness
- manipulation
- rehabilitation to increase movement and flexibility
- education about preventing back pain and taking care of the back.

One of the difficulties in judging the success of any physical type of therapy is that any treatment which involves the practitioner examining and touching the sufferer's body and active listening, has a very powerful effect in making that person feel better. This 'placebo effect' arises from the benefits of the human touch and care rather than the actual treatment given. When a physical therapy is compared with a non-touch treatment, such as a course of tablets, the placebo effect resulting from the physical therapy may be greater than that from the course of tablets, making it difficult to compare the two.

Summary of evidence to date

Medication[22]

- Paracetamol or non-steroidal anti-inflammatory drugs (NSAIDs) or paracetamol-weak opioid compounds (codydramol or coproxamol) should be prescribed at regular intervals to control pain, rather than be taken as necessary.
- Muscle relaxants effectively reduce acute back pain, but they do have side effects of drowsiness and potential physical dependence even after courses as short as a week.
- Strong opioids such as morphine and pethidine appear no more effective than safer analgesics in relieving low back pain.
- NSAIDs prescribed at regular intervals give effective pain relief in simple acute backache. Ibuprofen, followed by diclofenac, has the lowest risk of gastrointestinal complications.
- NSAIDs are more effective than paracetamol for overall improvement and more effective than placebo for pain relief.[20]
- Antidepressants are widely used for chronic low back pain, although there is little evidence for their effectiveness and none for their use in acute back pain.
- Trigger point and ligamentous injections: there is limited evidence of their effectiveness in chronic back conditions and little evidence in acute back pain.
- Epidural steroid injections, with or without local anaesthetic, produce better short-term relief of acute back pain with sciatica than comparable treatments.
- Facet joint injections do not appear to reduce pain or improve chronic back pain, and there is no evidence of efficacy in acute back pain.

Topical treatments

It is known that topical NSAIDs are more effective than placebo creams in relieving acute pain conditions. However, the relative advantages of topical NSAIDs over paracetamol are not known.[20]

Physical therapies and exercise[22]

- There is strong evidence that bed rest may lead to debilitation, chronic disability and increasing difficulty in rehabilitation.

- Continuing ordinary, everyday activities leads to the most speedy recovery and least time off work; a planned return to normal work within a short time leads to less time off work in the long run.
- Psychosocial factors influence response to treatment and rehabilitation.
- Manipulation provides short-term improvement in pain and activity for acute and subacute back pain; risks of complications are low.
- Exercise programmes can improve pain and functioning in people with chronic low back pain. There is no evidence that specific back exercises such as aerobic or strengthening exercises are more effective than other conservative treatments in acute low back pain.
- Acupuncture may reduce pain and increase activity in people with chronic back pain.
- Biofeedback: there is conflicting evidence on the effectiveness of biofeedback in chronic back pain, and none in acute back pain.

Ice, heat and massage may all be used for relieving symptoms of pain and stiffness of the back, but do not appear to have any effect on speeding up recovery.

An icepack can be made from crushed ice or a packet of frozen peas. Prevent an ice burn by applying baby oil to bare skin or wearing light clothing, and wrapping the ice or frozen peas in a tea towel. The icepack should be held against the painful area of the back (or any other painful part of the body) for a minimum of five, but preferably a maximum of ten, minutes. If symptoms are relieved repeat this treatment three times a day.

There is no scientific evidence confirming the effectiveness of traction for acute or chronic low back pain or nerve root problems, but it is commonly used by therapists for symptom relief alongside other treatment methods.

Traction is set up by passing a strap across the chest and another around the pelvis. While the chest strap is fixed, a weight is applied to the strap around the pelvis, pulling the spine to its full length and so relieving pressure on the intervertebral discs. Traction is generally applied for between 15 and 20 minutes as an outpatient; the treatment might be repeated up to three times a week for a number of weeks. Inpatients have weights attached to the legs, often for long periods.

Electrical therapies[22]

These therapies appear to give useful relief of symptoms, but scientific evidence about the extent to which they speed recovery is inconclusive. Electrical therapies are given by different machines operated by a therapist. Not every therapist will be able to provide each type of therapy; because the evidence of their relative benefits is inconclusive, doctors and therapists tend to have their own preferences and beliefs as to what works best.

Ultrasound is thought to work by causing a reaction in the body's tissues that stimulates a healing response.

Short-wave diathermy creates an electromagnetic field in the body's tissues, which alternates direction rapidly and can produce heat. It is usually given in a pulsed form so that the heating effect does not occur. Its effect is thought to be mediated through an alteration in the charges on cell membranes, establishing a more normal state in the tissues.

Interferential therapy is given as two currents of varying frequency passed through the body's tissues. Stimulating those tissues is thought to create an increase in blood flow and reduction in pain transmission.

Laser therapy using light waves is thought to stimulate healing in soft tissues.

Transcutaneous electrical nerve stimulation (TENS) relieves symptoms rather than influences the speed of recovery from either acute or chronic low back pain.[20] TENS is thought to block the transmission of pain impulses along sensory nerves to the brain. Most people use a . TENS machine for an hour at a time, giving them an ongoing effect for a few hours. A TENS machine is particularly useful when a person's choice of treatments for back pain is limited by their not being able to take drugs.

> A TENS machine is pocket-sized and can be operated by the person with pain. People using them are fully mobile. A TENS machine can be attached underneath clothing so that no-one knows you are wearing it.

Physical aids[22]

- Shoe insoles may reduce mild back pain in some people, but there is no evidence of long-term benefit.

- Lumbar corsets or supports: there is no evidence that these are effective in acute or chronic back pain.[20]

The evidence for complementary therapies

The common complementary therapies considered here are: acupuncture, manipulation, massage and aromatherapy, chiropractic, osteopathy, herbal medicine and homeopathy.

> 40% of general practices provide access to some form of complementary therapy; 25% of practices make NHS referrals to complementary therapies.[28]

Some complementary practitioners are practising health professionals, such as doctors, physiotherapists or nurses who are state registered with their own professional bodies. Others such as osteopaths and chiropractors, are registered with their own statutory bodies and accountable to those bodies for the standards of their practice. Patients can seek legal redress in the event of something going wrong. Other complementary practitioners who are not currently subject to statutory regulation may be so in future. Most complementary practitioners have completed further education in their discipline, even if they can legally practise without any training. Many therapists belong to registering or accrediting bodies of their own organisations; contact details are given at the back of this book.

It is becoming increasingly difficult to distinguish between what might be regarded as 'conventional' NHS treatment and 'alternative' therapies, as some practitioners offer both approaches, and some traditional 'alternative' therapies such as aromatherapy and acupuncture are readily available as an integral part of NHS care in some areas of the UK.

Many complementary practitioners aim to restore balance to the body and facilitate the body's own healing responses rather than target specific symptoms or diseases. Many conventional health professionals practise in this holistic manner too, relating treatment to the whole person, including their physical, psychological, social and spiritual states. Sometimes therapists use more than one treatment in combination.

Acupuncture

Acupuncture originated in China and has been practised for more than 5000 years. Acupuncture points run along 'meridian' channels. Needles are inserted into specific, designated points on the body relating to particular sites of pain suffered by the patient or client. Stimulation from the needle points redirects channels of energy beneath the skin to restore the body's energy levels (called *qi* or *chi*) and create 'harmony' in the normal bodily functions. Acupuncture considers the whole body rather than concentrating solely on specific symptoms, as Western medicine tends to do. A minority of doctors and therapists working for the NHS have trained in acupuncture. Training might vary from a two-day weekend course to many years of intensive study. Some spend time in China, where acupuncture is a routine method of providing pain relief and treating many other conditions, learning and practising their techniques according to the Chinese culture.

The usual 'Western' approach is to insert a few fine needles (perhaps three or four) for around 20 minutes or so; with the Chinese approach, needles may be left in for up to one hour. The needles may be rotated in the skin by the practitioner to restimulate the acupuncture point. Disposable needles are usually used; they are reasonably cheap, costing the acupuncturist a few pence at a time. The number of treatment sessions depends on the response and the practitioner's usual practice.

Complications from acupuncture are rare, but include puncturing the lung so that air is sucked in, creating a pneumothorax, bleeding from the needle sites and, occasionally, worsening of pain after the initial session.

Acupuncturists with the letters 'MBAcC' after their name are registered by the British Acupuncture Council; practitioners qualified as doctors might be members of the British Medical Acupuncture Society (BMAS), and some doctors and physiotherapists may simply describe themselves by their professional qualifications (for example MB BS; MCSP or SRP respectively).

'Weak and equivocal evidence suggests that acupuncture may reduce pain and enable increased activity in patients with chronic low back pain. There is no evidence of efficacy of acupuncture for acute low back problems'.[22] One of the problems of establishing how effective acupuncture is, is that different acupuncturists use different techniques. They vary as to the sites of the body, lengths of time needles are left in and whether they attach small electric currents to the needles (electro-acupuncture). Few research studies have followed up study patients for long enough to be able to measure longer-term outcomes.

A meta-analysis of randomised controlled trials of acupuncture for back pain concluded that acupuncture was superior to various other control interventions; but four sham-controlled, evaluator-blinded studies did not show acupuncture to be superior to placebo.[29]

Another alternative way of delivering an acupuncture effect is by acupoint stimulation. This may be self-administered via an electric stimulator through an acupuncture point; electric stimulators are sold directly to the public from some chemist shops and through mail order.

Acupressure is exerted by finger pressure to acupuncture sites. It is not thought to be as powerful as using acupuncture needles and the benefit may be more like that from deep massage. The acupressure is sometimes applied through fixing a plant seed on the skin, or using a pencil point or magnetic balls.

Manipulation

An overview of the evidence reports that there is 'conflicting evidence about the effects of spinal manipulation in acute and chronic low back pain'.[20] Other guidelines recommend that 'manipulation provides better short-term improvement in pain and activity levels and higher patient satisfaction than other treatments to which it has been compared in acute and subacute back pain'.[22] It is impossible to predict exactly who will respond and when, or what kind of manipulation is most effective in relieving pain or increasing spinal movement.

Different forms of spinal manipulation are practised by various therapists; physiotherapists, osteopaths, chiropractors and some medical practitioners tend to favour their own specialty's way of performing manipulation. The therapist employs various skills and techniques with his or her hands on the spine. The range of manipulation procedures varies from massage to high velocity thrusts and includes: long-lever, non-specific manipulation; specific, short-lever, high-velocity spinal adjustments; active or functional manipulation; mobilisation; manual traction; soft tissue massage; and point pressure manipulation. Manipulation seems to be most effective in people with acute low back pain without leg pain or neurological deficits. It appears to increase the spinal range of movement. There are few risks from manipulation for low back pain, provided that patients are selected and assessed properly and it is carried out by a trained therapist or practitioner.

> Manipulation should not be used in patients with symptoms that include: cancer, pregnancy, severe or progressive neurological symptoms, osteoporosis, where the back pain is originating from other parts of the body than the spine, or ankylosing spondylitis, as it might potentially cause a worsening of the symptoms or even a fracture if the manipulated spine was osteoporotic.

Chiropractic

Chiropractic treatment for back pain involves mechanical manipulation of the spine. Chiropractors manipulate the vertebrae by sharp thrusts with their hands on the spine. In one study in 1998, 3% of adults with back pain in the UK had consulted a chiropractor in the previous year.[28]

> One research trial comparing chiropractic manipulation treatment with hospital therapists using their normal range of treatment, including Maitland mobilisation or manipulation techniques, found that 'for patients with low back pain in whom manipulation is not contraindicated, chiropractic manipulation almost certainly confers worthwhile, long-term benefit in comparison with hospital outpatient management. The benefit was seen mainly in those with chronic or severe pain.' The people with back pain who received chiropractic manipulation in this trial were still more satisfied with the outcome three years later compared to those who received the hospital-based treatments.[30] Publication of this study produced a flurry of critical correspondence pointing out the lack of validity from comparing the results of private and unhurried sessions of chiropractic treatment with those from the average overworked and understaffed NHS physiotherapy unit.

Aromatherapy and massage, including Shiatsu, Reiki and Rolfing

Many powers have been attributed to fragrant plants and they have long been used in the pursuit of health. Each plant has a characteristic aroma and flavour because of its essential oils. The oil may be extracted from the flowers, leaves, fruit, stems, wood, bark, resin or roots. Aromatherapy oils might be added as a few drops to a bath, or used as a massage blend, a perfume, an inhalant, a compress, a vapouriser or a room spray. The effects are exerted as the oil is absorbed through the skin and into the bloodstream, and by the aroma being breathed in to work on the person's psychological state and emotions.

In Britain, two types of aromatherapy are used. 'Aesthetic' aromatherapy is carried out as a general treatment at beauty clinics and health farms to create a feeling of wellbeing, whereas 'holistic' aromatherapy is carried out by trained professionals to treat specific disorders. A holistic approach in aromatherapy is about treating the 'whole' person rather than narrowing down on specific symptoms or health problems.

Marjoram oil, basil and ginger are all thought to relieve muscular discomfort and fatigue; other oils, such as jasmine and vetivert, are relaxing and may help soothe back pain.

The practice of massage is a universal concept of healing. The manipulation of the body's soft tissues through stroking, rubbing, kneading and tapping increases circulation, improves muscle tone, and relaxes the body and mind. Massage is described as having other therapeutic effects: as a cleanser by stimulating lymph circulation and accelerating the elimination of wastes and toxins; by dilating blood vessels to improve the circulation, nutrition of the tissues and relieve congestion throughout the body; by relieving tension and relaxing muscle spasms.

There are various forms of massage, including Swedish, Shiatsu, Reiki and Rolfing techniques. In Swedish massage, the therapist usually starts on the back, working down to the legs, then, when the client turns over, the chest, abdomen, shoulders and face are treated. This type of massage is the one usually practised in sports centres and health clubs.

Shiatsu is the oldest documented form of physical therapy, dating back to 500BC. It is a type of oriental massage, which concentrates on particular points of the body rather than the whole body to rebalance the flow of *chi* in the body, thought to be 'life energy' that circulates around the body in channels. The palms and thumbs are used to apply pressure to the skin at places that often correspond to acupoints. It is possible that Shiatsu therapy acts like acupuncture, stimulating certain meridians and the body to help itself. Normally clients lie on a futon (Japanese floor mattress) for the treatment.

Reiki involves touch therapy, through the practitioner's hands being placed on parts of the body near the site of the problem, such as the back, to encourage energy flows through the therapist's hands to the patient. Sessions last for about an hour.

Rolfing aims to rebalance the body by bringing the head, shoulders, chest, pelvis and legs into proper vertical alignment so that the recipient feels more supple and musculoskeletal problems such as bad backs improve incidentally. The therapy usually consists of at least ten sessions focused on different parts of the body. The therapist applies pressure with his or her fingers, hands, knuckles or elbows to lengthen and release the connective tissues of different sites of the body. It can be a painful therapy.

Most massage sessions last between 30 and 90 minutes.

Osteopathy

Osteopathy was the first complementary therapy to be regulated by law in the UK in 1993. Diagnosis and assessment precedes physical manipulation of ligaments, bones, joints and muscles to relieve pain, improve movement and enhance health. Osteopaths use their hands to stretch soft tissues and mobilise joints through rhythmic passive movements and high-velocity thrust techniques, to improve mobility and the range of joint movement. Treatment is often accompanied by an audible 'click'. Six per cent of UK adults with back pain visited an osteopath in 1998, compared to 10% who visited a physiotherapist.[17]

Homeopathy

Homeopathy is based on the principle that a little of what makes a person worse can make a person better, so that substances that in large doses will cause the symptoms of an illness can be used in minute quantities to relieve the same symptoms. Half of all homeopathic treatments are bought over-the-counter from shops and pharmacies, and half are prescribed by homeopathic practitioners. Some are branded medicines and others are flower remedies. The ailments for which homeopathic medicines are bought are wide-ranging, and include coughs and colds, digestive complaints, skin conditions and joint pains.

Some homeopathic practitioners use formica (the sting of ants) and acus mould (the sting of honey bees) for injections into joints as an alternative to steroid injections. The sting is diluted many times, but may still trigger a reaction to the venom, which is thought to stimulate a healing effect.

Homeopathic medicines with a wide spectrum of activity are called *polychrests*; while *complex* remedies are a mixture of medicines, usually with specific uses. Homeopathic remedies may be given as tablets, granules or powders.

Homeopathic remedies are used in a diluted form and are not addictive. The numbers after the names indicate the extent of dilution; 6c is generally recommended for ailments that have developed over a longer period of time, whereas the stronger 30c is generally used for acute conditions. Potentially toxic concentrations of some homeopathic drugs have been described, and occasional allergic reactions.

Examples of homeopathic medicines that are recommended for various forms of back pain include: acetic acid 12, aconite 12, aesculus 12, aloe 12, bryonia 12, calc fluor 12, chelidonium 12, cimicifuga 12, gnaphalium 12, hydrastis 12, kali carb 12, kali phos 12, ledum 12, nux vom 12, rhus tox 12, ruta 12 and sepia 12. A homeopathic practitioner would specify which type of treatment was appropriate for different sites and descriptions of pain and weakness, and would prescribe treatment until improvement occurred. Side effects are more likely with more concentrated doses and include: laxative (e.g. bryonia), gastric irritant or abortion (e.g. ledum) and heart failure (e.g. aconite).

There is currently no single registering body. Those homeopaths who are registered with the Society of Homeopaths must hold professional insurance and have passed academic and clinical assessments.

Herbal medicines

Herbal medicines are made from roots, flowers, bark or plant extracts. People who treat themselves with herbal preparations may mistakenly assume that these products are safe because they are 'natural', but they can have adverse effects either when taken alone or from interactions with prescription medications. They are commonly taken for sleeplessness, listlessness, and general aches and pains, and so may be tried for back pain.

Herbal medicines are not subject to such strict controls as regulated pharmaceutical medicines, and some can be contaminated by other substances. Although serious contamination is rare, there have been two cases reported in the UK recently where the patients died from kidney failure after taking contaminated herbal preparations for their eczema; and more than 100 Belgian patients have recently been reported to have suffered kidney damage from Chinese herb preparations.

Herbal remedies are not usually prescribed for single diseases, but for generalised conditions. Some examples of herbal preparations that might be used for general muscular and bony aches and pains or back pain in particular are:

- St John's Wort, which may be used for treating musculoskeletal pain. It is an extract from the hypericum bush. The effect might be mediated through improving underlying anxiety and/or depression. Side effects are photosensitivity and cataracts.
- glucosamine sulphate, which is regarded as a 'food for cartilage' in that it is thought to stimulate production of cartilage components and allow rebuilding of damaged cartilage. Glucosamine is usually taken as 1.5 g per day as an oral dose or as an injection of 400 mg two or three times per week. Side effects are few but if they do occur include: mild stomach pain, heartburn, drowsiness, diarrhoea and nausea.

> Several research trials have shown that glucosamine is effective for arthritis pain. It is as effective as taking 1.2 g per day of the NSAID ibuprofen, at least in the short term.[31]

- red pepper extract – topical capsicum or black pepper – known as 'substance P'. This is used for joint pains. It is taken continuously rather than as an ad hoc treatment. Adverse reactions are dose- and concentration-dependent. They include: eye symptoms, burning pain in nose or sneezing, cough, skin irritation and gastric discomfort.
- celery seeds, which have been used to relieve rheumatic pains. Adverse effects include: sedation, dermatitis and a tendency to allergic reactions. Consumption in quantities greater than that contained in food are not recommended by some experts.

We do not fully understand how many herbal medicines work. With their growing popularity, GPs and pharmacists should be more alert to the possibility that a patient or customer is taking a herbal medicine and bear in mind potential herb–drug interactions.[32]

Mental therapies

The extent to which people recover from their first acute episode of back pain and the likelihood of it recurring depends very much on their state of health before the onset of back pain and how they maintain their health afterwards.

Pain can dominate a person's whole life and make them depressed and apathetic. They may feel that they have lost control over their life and cease to struggle to overcome the pain. Back pain may keep them awake at night so that chronic tiredness compounds their low mood and negativity. Some complementary therapies that are used for their effects on the mind are: autogenic training, hypnosis, meditation, naturopathy, relaxation and visualisation, and yoga.

General dissatisfaction with life and work influence whether low back pain persists, as well as low mood and social withdrawal described as 'yellow flags' on page 24. Any mental therapies that tackle these conditions may have a secondary effect on improving back pain. People's beliefs or behaviours play a key role in predicting the likelihood of their getting better.

Some studies show that acute low back pain is reduced by practising relaxation, others that chronic pain is lessened to the same extent as using other non-medical methods. The benefits of relaxation may lie in its ability to make people feel better rather than to relax muscles and relieve pain.

Hypnotherapy

Therapists usually induce a deeply relaxed state by hypnosis, and may then make therapeutic suggestions to relieve symptoms.

Self-hypnosis has been used as a way of helping people with severely disabling low back pain to cope more adequately with their pain problem, rather than to reduce the actual intensity of the back pain.

There are over 100 different types of complementary or alternative therapies. Besides those already described above, others that have been tried for back pain and back problems include: water therapy, iridology, crystal therapy and T'ai chi.

Treatments that are likely to be harmful[22]

It is worth trying a new therapy if others haven't been successful. But for some treatments there is evidence that potential hazards or complications pose too great a risk and they should not be tried. Those that should be avoided include:

- bed rest with or without traction, as neither is effective and may create such complications as pressure sores, thromboembolism and joint stiffness
- manipulation under general anaesthetic, which may cause serious neurological damage
- applying a plaster jacket, as it may cause sores from rubbing, spinal stiffness, muscle wasting and breathing problems
- steroid drugs, as there are complications with longer than short-term use
- relaxants such as diazepam, to which people may become easily addicted.

Who should do what in your practice or pharmacy team?

The GP

The GP's main role is to provide effective clinical management for those with back pain and take ultimate responsibility for the efficient organisation of practice systems so that patients can access and receive best practice in clinical management.

The GP might write the practice protocol based on national guidelines[22,23] with other team members' input and agreement, then undertake or delegate systematic audits of the guidelines to gauge the extent to which clinical staff adhere to the guidelines, organising education and training if appropriate.

The GP is required under the NHS Terms of Service to provide advice to his or her patients about whether, as a result of a medical disease or disablement (e.g. back pain), the patient should refrain from their usual type of work.

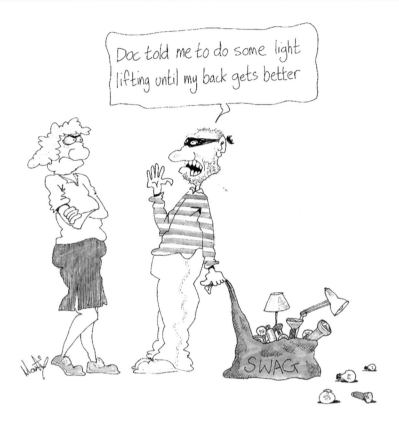

The pharmacist

The pharmacist's main role is to advise the person with back pain (or their family, if consulting on the person's behalf) about self-care, pain relief, side effects of medication and drug interactions, appropriate referral to the GP or complementary practitioners, and sale of supportive equipment and over-the-counter remedies.

1 Advising on self-care, the main messages being that:
   • pain does not equal harm
   • bed rest makes the condition worse
   • getting back to normal activities leads to an earlier recovery
   • people who are physically fit generally get less back pain and recover faster if they do get back pain.
2 Providing pain relief, including conventional treatments, herbal and homeopathic remedies, or topical NSAIDs.
3 Warning of and avoiding side effects of medication and drug interactions, such as advising that paracetamol is tried before

NSAIDs are taken, and drawing customers' attention to risks of NSAIDs.

4 Referring to GPs if there is a suspicion of 'red flags', there is a need for pain relief or back pain is persisting. Referring to others, such as complementary practitioners, as appropriate.

5 Sale of supportive equipment as appropriate.

Community nurse

The roles of nurses and health visitors working in primary care include:

- advising patients and clients with back pain about self-care and pain relief
- looking after their own backs and those of their colleagues. Nurses and health visitors are at risk of injuring their own backs while lifting and handling patients or equipment. Nurses typically develop back injuries from manual handling, but pre-existing problems can be aggravated by car journeys or sitting on floors and in uncomfortable chairs in clients' homes while providing nursing care
- noting obvious interactions with the patient's current medication and not so obvious interactions with other over-the-counter (OTC) drugs, including complementary therapies that the patient does not necessarily volunteer that he or she is taking
- suggesting appropriate referral to the GP, complementary practitioner or pharmacist for OTC remedies. A community nurse or health visitor should know the location of the main providers of healthcare, including complementary therapists. They should be confident that those whom they recommend to people with back pain have valid professional or specialty qualifications. Reasons for advising patients to see their GPs will include any suspicion of symptoms or signs that indicate 'red flag' conditions, persistent back pain or back problems limiting function, or inadequacy of OTC medication in relieving symptoms.

Physical therapist

The therapist's role is to provide appropriate physical care to patients with back pain. Studies exploring the placebo effect of physical therapy highlight the care and compassion therapists exude in their close, touching relationships with patients.

The therapist should communicate news of the patient's progress to the referring health professionals and other team members as appropriate. Then re-refer the patient back to the GP if progress is less good than expected or sinister symptoms present.

Reflection exercises

Exercise 5 (for GPs and pharmacists). Compose a practice or pharmacy protocol

Or draw up advice sheets for people with back pain, if you do not already have a protocol or advisory literature. You will need to include the information from these first three chapters, basing your material on the evidence for what works:

1 Initial assessment: the patient should be classified as to whether they have:
   - simple backache (non-specific low back pain)
   - nerve root pain
   - possible serious spinal pathology, termed 'red flags'
   - psychosocial symptoms and signs termed 'yellow flags'.
2 Medication:
   - pain relief should be prescribed regularly, rather than as required
   - appropriate analgesia
   - avoid medication with potential adverse effects as far as possible; for example, NSAIDs and muscle relaxants reduce acute back pain effectively but have potentially serious adverse effects, so paracetamol is safer as the first line drug.
3 Appropriate activities:
   - do not prescribe bed rest as a treatment for simple back pain
   - advise patients to continue normal activities and gradually increase activities over a short period of days or weeks
   - if the patient is in work, advise them to stay at work if at all possible. Urge return to work as soon as possible
   - consider alternative or complementary therapies if patients need additional help with their pain during the first six weeks.
4 X-ray only if appropriate:[26]
   - straight lumbar–sacral X-rays should not be organised for acute low back problems within six weeks of the onset of symptoms unless a 'red flag' is noted
   - X-ray if appropriate for patient history or findings.

5 Referral for specialist help:
   • for persistent nerve root pain
   • possible serious spinal pathology
   • suspected cauda equina syndrome.
6 Active rehabilitation for those having difficulty returning to normal working at approximately 4–12 weeks will include:
   • education directed at managing pain and overcoming disability
   • reassurance and advice: to stay active
   • an active and progressive exercise and fitness programme
   • pain management using behavioural principles
   • the patient being directed strongly towards return to work
   • symptomatic relief measures should support and not interfere with rehabilitation.

Exercise 6 (for GPs, pharmacists and community nurses). Undertake an audit of your advice to people with back pain

Compare your performance against best practice for self-care, pain relief, side effects of medication and drug interactions, appropriate referral to GP or complementary practitioners.

Keep a record of the advice given to the next ten patients who consult you about their back pain. Photocopy this page and complete a page for each person who consults you with back pain. Then check how this matches current best practice as described earlier.

1 Did you advise the patient to stay as active as possible, and continue normal activities?

       Yes   No   Not applicable

2 Was the patient advised to stay at work?

       Yes   No   Not applicable

3 Did you advise against bed rest?

       Yes   No

4 Did you advise that, for most back problems, pain does not mean that the spine is being damaged?

       Yes   No

5 Did you recommend that the patient controlled the pain with paracetamol as an initial treatment?

> Yes   No

6 If you recommended that the patient controlled the pain with NSAIDs, did you check for contraindications to NSAIDs and warn of potential side effects?

> Yes   No

7 Did you check whether the person with back pain was taking alternative oral therapies already, before dispensing a prescription or recommending an analgesic?

> Yes   No

8 Did you give advice about exercise and keeping physically fit?

> Yes   No

9 Did you give the person with back pain or his/her representative any literature about self-care?

> Yes   No

Conclude: are you managing and treating patients in accordance with recommended best practice? Have you any learning needs?

Exercise 7 (for GPs, pharmacists, community nurses and therapists)

You might meet together as a local general medical practice team and run a multidisciplinary learning session around the management of back pain. The preparation you do prior to the event and the discussion at the practice meeting will show you some of your weaknesses and therefore learning needs.

> **Conclude**: what you need to learn to be able to give people with back pain advice about self-care, medication, clinical management, investigations, occupational advice and OTC treatments that equate with best practice.

Exercise 8 (for GPs). Complete this case study[33] of appropriate sickness certification of a patient with back pain

A 42-year-old woman has worked as a hotel receptionist for many years. She has recurrent episodes of low back pain and is frequently 'off work' for four to eight weeks. Her employers are finding it increasingly difficult to cope with her prolonged and frequent absences. A week previously, while digging the garden she developed low back pain which did not radiate to her legs. She has complained that bending is painful and that she is more comfortable if she is able to change position from time to time. She has spent long periods resting in bed, as in the past she has been advised that bed rest is the best treatment for back pain; this, however, has produced no improvement in her symptoms. Otherwise she is well. On examination, she has an almost full range of back movements with no neurological signs in her legs.

She requests a certificate. Should you issue a certificate advising this woman to refrain from work and what are the possible consequences of your action?

(This exercise is reproduced by kind permission of Dr Philip Sawney, Department of Social Security.)[33]

Write your answer first and then look at page 55 for a suggested response.

Answer to case study of appropriate sickness certification of a patient with back pain[33,34]

Before you complete the Med 3 certificate choosing between 'I have examined you today and advised you that you need not/should refrain from work' you should:

- explore the patient's expectations and motivation to work
- determine the nature of the patient's condition: is it simple back pain, or is there evidence of nerve compression or sinister back pain (see Chapter 2)
- find out if she has functional limitations in relation to the tasks she performs at work
- consider if there is anything that might be done at work to enable the patient to continue working. This might involve liaison with the occupational health service at her place of work if there is such a service, reasonable adjustments under the Disability Discrimination Act 1995 or reasonably practicable precautions under the Health and Safety at Work Act 1974 or the Manual Handling Regulations (see Chapter 5)
- compare your management of this woman with national guidelines on back pain management.[22,23] There are a range of treatments with evidence to support them that you might try – as described in the guidelines
- withstanding pressure to meet the patient's expectations of a sickness certificate and encouraging her positive attitude to work may be hard, but in her long-term best interests. More appropriate clinical management may enable this patient to continue at work. There are many social and financial benefits to being at work, as well as continuing normal activities being key to best practice in simple back pain management. Issuing a sickness certificate may undermine the patient's ability to overcome potentially incapacitating symptoms; it will be likely to lead to requests for further certificates in the future and may cause financial problems for the patient
- involving the patient in decision making about her clinical management will include exploring her expectations, explaining best practice, seeking her permission to liaise with her employer and occupational health services about altering her working environment or actual job if that is appropriate.

Now, take another case of your own; a patient with back pain where you have vacillated over whether or not the patient's condition warranted you issuing a sickness certificate in response to the patient's request. Analyse what happened in that case, what the outcome was and whether you acted in the patient's best interests in the longer term.

Conclude: do you need to brush up on your knowledge of sickness certification and could you usefully study the Department of Social Security's Guide for GPs?[34] Do you need to learn more about assertiveness skills?[35] Are you advising patients with acute or chronic back pain about continuing at work in line with guidelines for best practice?

Exercise 9 (for GPs, pharmacists, nurses and therapists). List all the providers in your neighbourhood of complementary therapies or treatments of whom you are aware

List them by their specialty (e.g. aromatherapy, osteopathy, chiropractic). Indicate if treatment is available on the NHS. Tick if you have their contact details easily to hand so that you can tell patients where they might seek help or advice. Indicate if you know whether they have state registered qualifications or other valid professional qualifications.

Providers of complementary therapies or treatments

Practice by specialty	Available on the NHS?	Tick if state registered qualification or equivalent	Tick if contact details easily to hand

Conclude: whether you need to find out more about alternatives to conventional NHS management. Do you need to learn more about the evidence base for various treatments or the validity of alternative practitioners' qualifications? Does the NHS provide these treatments? For instance, a practice nurse might be trained in aromatherapy, a physiotherapist might offer acupuncture. It is also worth finding out relative costs if treatments are only available privately.

Now that you have completed one or more of the interactive reflection exercises in this chapter, transfer the information from this needs assessment to the empty template of the PDP on pages 107–110 if you are working on your own learning plan; or to the practice PPDP on pages 133–136 if you are working on a practice-team learning plan. The conclusions made at the end of each exercise will feature in the action plan. Don't forget to keep evidence of your learning in your personal portfolio.

CHAPTER FOUR

Sensible advice about self-help for people in general and employees

Two photocopyable leaflets that give sensible advice about self-care are included in Appendix 3 for you to distribute to people with back pain and back problems. These self-help leaflets are an abbreviated version of the material in this chapter.

In 1995, the general public in the UK spent an estimated £1.24 billion on OTC products for symptom relief. These included conventional treatments, some of which are also available through a doctor's prescription, and alternatives such as homeopathic therapies or herbal medicines.[19]

Self-care, prescribed and alternative therapies are not mutually exclusive; one is sometimes used to complement another, so that adding different types together can achieve more effective control of symptoms.

The key messages[36,37] are that:

- pain does not equal harm
- bed rest makes back pain worse
- back pain is usually not due to anything serious
- getting back to normal activities leads to an earlier recovery
- people who are physically fit generally get less back pain and recover faster if they do get back pain.

People can do a great deal themselves to help their backs withstand the stresses and strains of everyday living and work, through exercise, activity and better posture. And reviewing the home environment, work or household chores should guard against triggering back pain through awkward lifting or avoidable accidents.

Exercises to prevent back problems in general

Remind patients not to become overweight and to take regular exercise doing something that they enjoy, such as swimming or walking for 20–30 minutes two or three times a week. They should build up the amount of exercise gradually to keep the spinal muscles in shape. The main advice is to remain as active as possible and continue normal daily activities.

> Exercise classes led by a physiotherapist that included strengthening exercises for all main muscle groups, stretching exercises, a relaxation session and brief education on back care, did help people suffering from mechanical back pain up to a year later. In Sweden, back classes run as 'back schools' in different work settings have been found to be effective in educating groups of workers about avoiding back pain.[38]

Exercises for a 'slipped disc'

If the pain is in the middle of the back, the sufferer will need to lean backwards; if it is on the left, they will need to squash down the left side of the spine in order to push the disc back into the middle of the vertebra and lean to the left. This may be the opposite of what seems natural: many people feel it is more comfortable to lean away from the painful side or to slouch in a chair, as these postures relieve pressure on the nerve roots. However such temporary relief helps to keep the disc out of position and delays recovery.

Every hour for the first two days, ten movements should be done to try to move the disc back into position. After this, the frequency of the exercise can be reduced, until a maintenance session once a day should be sufficient to prevent further problems when the back has settled down.

If the pain is in the centre of the lumbar spine, the sufferer should lie on the floor with their hands under their shoulders and push up until their arms are straight, leaving their hips on the floor. At the ninth or tenth movement, they should try to relax the muscles around the lumbar spine so that their hips sag to the floor. Lying on their front for periods of 15–20 minutes, such as while watching television or reading, may be useful. If there are neck problems too, or it is difficult or inconvenient to get down on the floor, the person can stand astride (standing upright with legs straight and feet apart by 50 cm [18″] or so) and lean backwards ten times with the hands on the waist.

With one-sided pain spreading into the buttock or leg, the sufferer should try to compress the painful side, by standing with legs apart beside a wall with the **painful** side **away from** the wall, resting the elbow against the wall and then gliding the hips in towards the wall ten times. The pain should usually lessen, or move upwards and towards the centre of the back. If this standing exercise doesn't help the pain, lying face down in the push-up position making a sideways kink in the spine with hips shifted **away from** the painful side and doing ten push-ups leaving hips on the floor, may do.

If neither of these exercises helps, rotating the spine may be the answer. They should lie on their back with knees bent and roll their knees over towards the painful side, leaving them there for two or three minutes and then returning to the centre again. This manoeuvre should be repeated three or four times.

Sometimes as the exercise pushes the jelly back into the centre of the disc, the extra volume creates a temporary increase in pain. The patient should be reassured that this will settle, so long as the pain is moving **upwards** towards the centre of their spine. If the reverse happens, the patient should stop doing the exercises that are causing the pain and consult the treating physiotherapist or doctor to be reassessed. Sometimes people benefit from flexion exercises instead of the extension movements just described.

Keeping active

Keeping active is the key recommendation for beating back pain. This means doing normal everyday activities as opposed to sitting around resting or doing overstrenuous sport or exercises. As a person recovers from their back problems and continues with their exercises to stretch backwards, he or she can also strengthen the muscles which do this movement by lying on his or her front and lifting the head, hands and shoulders off the ground. The exercise can be made more difficult as the person becomes stronger by putting the hands under the forehead.

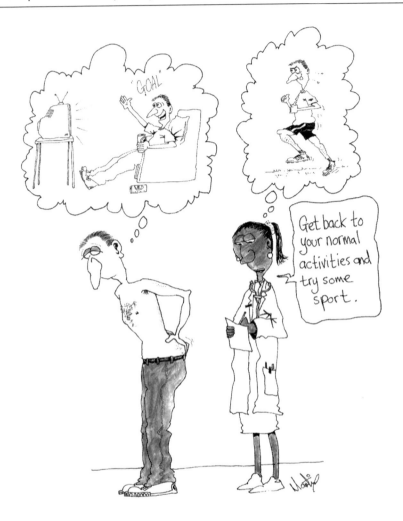

It is important to strengthen the abdominal muscles. These give support to the lumbar spine by pressing on the contents of the abdomen, using them to form a kind of splint along the spine, so that when lifting, any load is spread evenly along the whole of the lower back. The way to do abdominal exercises is to lie on the floor, bend the knees, preferably placing the calves on a stool, then lift the head to look at the knees. As people become stronger, they may be able to reach forwards and eventually to sit up. It is not advisable to do sit-ups by fixing the feet under furniture with legs out straight, as this puts a strain on the discs of the spine. There are also diagonal muscles to exercise, and reaching down to the outside of each opposite thigh will work these. The muscles at the side of the abdomen can be toned up by lying on one side and lifting the upper leg. Start with ten of each movement, gradually increasing the number every few days as strength increases.

Advice for people with back pain

- take care how you sit, drive, sleep, exercise, work, lift, and handle patients and equipment
- do not sit for too long at any one time, stand up and walk around regularly
- sit on firm chairs
- use simple painkillers
- sleep on a bed with a firm mattress – if the mattress is soft, put a board under it or put it on the floor
- walking and swimming are good exercises to prevent a recurrence of back pain; but swimming can aggravate acute back pain and is best avoided if pain is present

Lifting better

Anyone who is not confident that they can lift an object safely shouldn't lift it. It may be too heavy or awkward. There is always an alternative way to move it without risking injury to the back. Sometimes it is not a heavy weight that does the damage, but a seemingly easy lift done without much thought, especially if the muscles are tired. All lifting should be done with a 'straight back/bent knees' posture, keeping the object close to the body while lifting. The reason for keeping the back straight while lifting is to ensure that the lifted weight exerts less leverage on the spine.

Everybody should try to get into the habit of bending their knees rather than their back when they go to lift something, holding the object close in towards their body and avoiding twisting sideways at the same time as they lift.

There are some situations where someone may be particularly at risk of twisting at the same time as lifting, such as when putting shopping in the back of the car, reaching forwards with a weight in their arms.

Improving posture

In bed

It is best to lie on a reasonably firm mattress with the head and neck supported so that the spine remains as straight as possible. If the mattress is too soft or sags, the person will sink into it and the spine will curve; if it is too hard, the spine may become an unsupported bridge between the shoulders and hips. Sleeping on the front rather than the back can put extra strain on the neck. If the person you are advising has another condition that prevents them from lying flat, it may be necessary to adapt his or her posture, perhaps by raising one end of the bed. Some back pain sufferers have found benefits from a waterbed, but others report that a waterbed makes their symptoms worse.

Sitting position

Sitting upright, well back on the chair with a roll or small cushion in the low back gives the lumbar spine support. A 'lumbar roll' can be bought through local pharmacies; it has an adjustable elastic strap so it can be fixed to the chair at the right level. Similarly, a back pain sufferer might buy a 'Harley wedge' to sit on so that the pelvis is tilted into a better position. A 'backfriend' is another type of seat insert that is said to be orthopaedically and ergonomically designed to provide a well-positioned back curve to support the spine; it is a two-piece moulded seat with adjustable hinges. The head and neck should be supported if possible. Low chairs, sitting with legs straight out in front on the floor or in bed, or curling up in an armchair with legs tucked underneath should all be avoided.

Standing or walking

Advise back pain sufferers to try to keep upright and maintain the curves of their lumbar spine and neck. If the low back becomes flatter, there is a tendency to become round-shouldered, with the chin poking forwards. Placing equal weight on each foot, especially if standing in one position for a long time, will help, and those who have a standing job should adjust the height of their working surface if possible. Trying to avoid reaching or stretching too far and avoiding twisting from the waist by moving the feet to turn should help too. Backward bends can be used to vary the position if the person is generally in a static position at work.

Everyday activities

Many everyday activities can cause problems when done with a poor posture. Ironing, vacuum cleaning, dusting, making beds, cleaning baths, washing up, gardening, watching TV, shopping, lifting, cleaning windows and driving all need to be performed in a way that avoids excess strain on the spine.

Ironing

Adjust the height of the ironing board, keeping weight evenly on both feet. Using a steam setting requires a lighter pressure. Several short sessions are better than one lengthy one.

Vacuum cleaning

An upright cleaner means less bending than a cylinder, but it may be heavier to push around. Advise the person using a vacuum cleaner to get help moving large pieces of furniture and to avoid twisting their body.

Dusting/making beds/cleaning baths

Kneeling down to do these tasks creates less strain than bending the back.

Washing up

If the sink is too low, the washing-up bowl can be raised by placing an upturned bowl beneath it. Opening the cupboard under the sink and placing one foot on the bottom shelf keeps the back straight while washing up.

Gardening

A gardener should kneel whenever possible, using a kneeler or knee pads, rather than bend over, and take care not to jerk suddenly to pull plants out or twist or strain. Lighter tasks should be interspersed with heavy digging, using long-handled, lightweight tools. Moving or carrying several small loads is better than shifting one large one.

Watching TV/reading/sewing/knitting

It is best to sit directly in front of the TV. Advise back-pain sufferers to sit up straight, not to let their head droop when knitting, sewing or reading, and to get up and move around frequently.

Shopping

It is better to use a trolley rather than a basket, provided it does not have stiff wheels and the person is careful how they lift the goods out. Loads can be evened out by using two bags and holding one in each hand. High heels cause extra strain on joints by tipping the wearer forwards.

Cleaning windows

Advise back pain sufferers to use a proper set of steps and not to balance on a box or stretch out too far. Several short sessions are better than pushing to do the entire job in one go.

Driving

A wedge or thin cushion under the buttocks will raise the hips to a horizontal position if when sitting in a car seat the hips are lower than the knees. Use of a lumbar roll can maintain a good sitting position with a hollow in the back. Home-shopping catalogues are full of ideas for aids to maintain comfortable positions; one example is a revolving car seat which saves struggling out of a seat when getting in or out of the car.

Making the environment safer

Encourage people to review their home and work environments to make them safer:

- reduce chances of slipping (for example on a loose rug) or tripping over objects lying around
- look at chairs and furniture: replace old sagging chairs and beds, and desks and work surfaces that force them to adopt bad positions.

The employee's perspective of health and safety[39]

The types of action employees can take, with the support of their employer, to prevent back pain or reduce its recurrence are:

- doing the work in a different way to eliminate the risk activity
- modifying the job, equipment, workstation or process
- altering the job pattern, such as by rotation through a series of tasks, extending the job or introducing breaks in routine
- using different tools or mechanising tasks as appropriate.

The Health & Safety at Work etc. Act 1974 provides the basic legal framework to promote good health and safety standards. Employees as well as employers have responsibilities under the Act to be aware of and must abide by the legal requirements. The main aims of the Act are to:

- secure the health and safety of people at work
- protect others against health and safety risks from work activity
- control danger from articles and substances used at work.

Some key extracts from this legislation are given in Appendix 1.

The Management of Health and Safety at Work Regulations 1999 also apply to all employees as well as employers. These deal with all health and safety concerns based on the general principles of:

- risk assessment
- risk reduction
- risk monitoring
- the provision of appropriate information and training
- consultation with workers on relevant health and safety matters.

Employees should:

- comply with the instructions or training given to them by the employer relating to use of equipment, machinery, dangerous substances, transport, production means and safety devices
- report work situations that may reasonably be considered to be a serious and immediate danger to health and safety
- report to the employer any shortcomings in the protection arrangements for health and safety.

Employees and employers should work together to identify and reduce risks or potential problems. The table below describes the approaches they should take.

Employers should . . .	*Employees should . . .*
• *identify* the problem(s), the hazards and who may be affected	• help their employer identify the problem • inform their employer straight away if they have work-related symptoms which don't go away after a few days
• *generate* ideas	• co-operate and make suggestions
• *evaluate* alternative solutions	• co-operate in testing and trying out solutions
• *select* appropriate action	• give informed views about possible action
• *plan* for change, including the necessary resources – people, time, training, money	• be positive about training
• *implement* the improvement	• give support to the agreed improvement • stick to agreed changes in procedure
• *monitor* the results	• monitor procedures and systems and report problems
• *review* effectiveness of change or improvement and revise as necessary	• co-operate in providing information for the review

Reflection exercises

Exercise 10 (for everyone). Review your lifestyle and normal activities

1 How much exercise do you take each week? How does it compare with:
   - exercising for 20–30 minutes a day, e.g. walking?
   - taking part in sports activities such as badminton, squash, hockey, etc., each week?
   - swimming regularly?
   - doing heavy DIY jobs or gardening regularly?
2 Do you know what sports and leisure facilities there are within easy reach of your home or work?
3 How long is it since you changed the mattress of your bed?
4 Do you have a comfortable chair that gives good support to your back:
   - at your desk at work?
   - for writing on a desk or a table at home?
   - for relaxing at home?

Conclude: are there any changes you can make to your lifestyle that will prevent or minimise back pain?

Exercise 11 (for people who suffer from back pain). Chart your progress

Keep a weekly diary of when your back pain occurs, what you try to do to prevent or treat the pain and the outcomes. You may detect triggers and be able to deduce what helps or hinders your progress.

Date	Wk 1	Wk 2	Wk 3	Wk 4	Wk 5	Wk 6	Wk 7	Wk 8
Quality of sleep								
Pain* during day								
Pain* at work								
Pain* in bed								
Stiffness* when at home								
Stiffness* when at work								
Medicines: type(s) dose frequency								
Exercise: type frequency								
Normal activities								
Therapy: type frequency								
Other information								

* Note the severity of the back pain and stiffness and how long it lasts on a scale of 1–5: 1 = severe, 2= uncomfortable, 3 = tolerable for 50% of the time, 4 = tolerable all the time, 5 = good.

Exercise 12 (for employees). Undertake risk assessments of your workplace linked to the activities you do at work

(i) Visual display screen equipment in your practice or pharmacy

Complete the form for your display screen and workstation.

Display screen swivels and tilts easily   Yes/No
Keyboard can be tilted and is separate from the screen   Yes/No

Chair is stable   Yes/No
Chair is adjustable and can be positioned for comfort   Yes/No
Seat back is adjustable in both height and tilt   Yes/No
Footrest is available   Yes/No

Conclude: are there any changes you could make? If so, can you make these changes yourself or will you consult your manager?

(ii) Manual handling

Assess the lifting involved in your everyday job.

- Have you been trained in manual handling?   Yes/No
  - do you know what weight is reasonable for you
    to lift without harm: from the floor, waist height,
    above your head?   Yes/No
  - do you usually lift with bent knees?   Yes/No
- How do you usually manage if you have to move a
  heavy object at work:
  - do you refuse to lift it?   Yes/No
  - do you ask a colleague to help?   Yes/No
  - is there equipment to help?   Yes/No
  - if there is equipment do you know how to use it? Yes/No
  - do you try to shift the object without lifting it up? Yes/No
- How would you cope with:
  - person who has had a cardiac or respiratory arrest
    and is lying on the floor?
  - an unconscious patient lying on the floor?
  - a person who has fallen in a confined space?

Conclude: do you need further training in manual handling? If so, how will you arrange that?

For answers to the above, see the detailed information in Chapter 5.

CHAPTER FIVE

Establishing a healthy and safe working environment: looking after the backs of staff, patients and visitors to the premises

Responsibilities of employers cover a whole range of personal and management issues, statutory requirements in the area of health and safety, and legal responsibility to appoint competent people to advise on health and safety. Best practice in minimising back problems in your workplace is covered by applying the regulations that oblige all employers to maintain a healthy and safe working environment for staff and visitors:

- Management of Health and Safety at Work Regulations 1999
- Workplace (Health, Safety and Welfare) Regulations 1992
- Accident reporting and Reporting of Injuries, Diseases and Dangerous Occurrence Regulations (RIDDOR), 1995
- Manual Handling Operations Regulations 1992
- Health and Safety (First Aid) Regulations 1981
- Provision and Use of Work Equipment Regulations 1998
- Health and Safety (Display Screen Equipment) Regulations 1992
- Control of Substances Hazardous to Health Regulations 1999
- Disability Discrimination Act 1995.

An employer's duty with respect to health and safety of staff and patients is to make the workplace safe and without risks to the health of staff or visitors to the premises.

Risk assessment

Risk assessment entails evaluating the risks to the health of staff and patients in your practice or unit, and deciding on the action needed to minimise or eliminate those risks.

A hazard: something with the potential to cause harm
A risk: the likelihood of that potential to cause harm being realised

---

There are five steps to risk assessment:[14,40]

1 Look for and list the hazards.
2 Decide who might be harmed and how.
3 Evaluate the risks arising from the hazards and decide whether existing precautions are adequate or more should be done.
4 Record the findings.
5 Review the assessment from time to time and revise it if necessary.

A 'suitable and sufficient' risk assessment should enable the employer to identify and prioritise the measures that need to be taken by a competent person: health and safety information, training for employees, necessary health surveillance, any monitoring that needs to be carried out, procedures to follow in the event of serious or imminent danger.

The steps in an action plan for undertaking a risk assessment will lead you to:

1 Nominate a 'competent' person as the risk assessor or trainer.
2 Provide training for the risk assessor or trainer as appropriate.
3 Identify the tasks that require a manual handling assessment
   – prioritise where there are many tasks that might be assessed.
4 Decide which employees will require work-based training.
5 Assess the need for and type of manual handling aids required: involve the staff (and patients) in gauging ease of use, comfort and appropriateness.
6 Train employees: plan a schedule of training and updating; record details of training.
7 Establish which priorities will be tackled: review accident and sickness absence record, observe all areas of the practice or pharmacy, check use of equipment and aids, and staff commitment

to safe practice. Staff involved in patient-handling might develop their own specialist patient risk assessment form with which they are more likely to comply.

8 Update manual handling policy; review all health and safety policies annually.
9 Provide resources for the above.
10 Undertake a regular audit of all manual handling-related issues and activities: identify areas for improvement next year.
11 Investigate all reported manual handling-related accidents and near misses to detect problems at an early stage and enable the practice to respond promptly and comprehensively to complaints and negligence.

A competent person within the practice must:

- be sufficiently competent to carry out the work
- be given adequate time and adequate resources to carry out their functions
- have adequate decision-making authority

and should have a knowledge and understanding of:

- the work being assessed
- the principles of risk assessment and prevention of risk
- up-to-date health and safety measures
- identification of hazards at work

and should be able to:

- identify health and safety issues
- assess the need for action
- design, develop and implement strategies and plans
- check the effectiveness of these strategies and plans
- promote health, safety and welfare advances and good practices
- recognise their limitations and know when to call for others with specific skills and expertise.

Risk management

Risk management involves applying preventive and protective measures that follow risk assessment, including planning, organisation, control, monitoring and review.

The four stages in risk management[40] are to:

- identify the key risks and any triggers, encouraging staff to volunteer and discuss observed risks and adverse events
- analyse the risk – how common is it, are there patterns or trends, what impact does it have, does that impact matter, investigate high risk occurrences
- control the risk – what we can do about it, implement changes in practice as necessary, feedback to staff
- cost the risk – look at the cost of getting it right versus the cost of a risky outcome.

Sometimes managing or controlling one risk has the knock-on effect of creating new or greater risks elsewhere. If you do not have a grasp of the bigger picture, you can make things worse – and more risky. For instance, if you sprinkle salt on the path leading up to the surgery when it is icy to reduce the physical risk of patients falling down, you increase your financial risk of being held liable for someone actually slipping down.

Risk management in your practice or unit will involve:

- drawing up a health and safety policy statement if there are five or more employees, and making staff aware of the policy and arrangements
- identifying and assessing hazards in the workplace, such as from manual handling, and current control measures; improving those control mechanisms where necessary
- identifying people at risk, such as cleaners, lone receptionists (at risk of assault and injury); then informing, instructing, training and supervising staff in health and safety matters and risk management
- identifying and reducing organisational factors that predispose to risk
- ensuring that articles and substances are moved, stored and used safely
- ensuring that equipment is safe and that safe systems of work are set and followed
- providing adequate first aid resources
- supporting doctors and staff after traumatic events.

Health and safety

A practice with five or more staff must have a written health and safety policy. It is advisable for smaller practices to adopt the same standards. This written policy needs to be based on a thorough risk assessment covering all activities, clinical and non-clinical, and all areas of the building. All employees in the practice should have a basic understanding of health and safety issues. General medical and pharmacy practices are not absolved from the legal requirement to have a comprehensive first aid kit with someone appointed to take charge of it.

Pre-employment health screening will assess the extent to which an employee is capable of doing the proposed job and avoid risks of back injuries (in this instance) or other adverse effects on their health. Regular health surveillance of employees, where appropriate, should detect hazards at an early stage and offer an opportunity to avoid or minimise their effects.

The example of a model Health and Safety Statement given below should include what arrangements have been made to identify hazards to health and safety and assess and control risks. Describe who is responsible for the various tasks listed and at what intervals the policy should be reviewed and updated. It should be signed by the employer.

The statement should be displayed in the practice and a copy made available to staff.

General statement of Health and Safety policy[41]

It is the policy of this general practice/pharmacy to provide, maintain and ensure a safe and healthy workplace. Equipment and systems of work will be maintained and reviewed regularly. Such information, training and supervision will be provided as is necessary to enable staff to work safely and without undue risk to their health or the health of others. Responsibility for the health and safety of all other users of our premises and those who may be affected by our activities is accepted.

All employees should be aware of their responsibility under the Health and Safety at Work Act to co-operate with the practice health and safety policy. Allocation of specific duties, and arrangements for implementing this policy are detailed below.

Responsibilities

- Overall responsibility for health and safety _____
  (partner)
- Management and implementation of the policy _____
  (practice manager)
  and in his/her absence _____
- Health and Safety training _____
- Practice first aider _____

General arrangements

Accident reporting
- All accidents must be recorded in the
  Accident Book located: _____

First aid
- First aid box is located: _____
- Maintaining and stocking box is
  responsibility of: _____

Fire Safety
- Fire policy, procedures and escape routes are
  displayed: _____
  NB Escape routes must be kept clear at all times
- Fire alarms will be checked weekly by: _____
- Fire extinguisher locations: _____
- Fire extinguishers will be checked annually by: _____
  Fire practices will be held quarterly.

Electrical safety
- All portable electrical equipment must be
  checked before use by: _____
- Periodic checks of mains electrical
  equipment will be carried out at regular
  intervals by: _____

Waste disposal
- Arrangements have been made for the disposal
  of clinical waste with: _____
- And for non-clinical waste with: _____

Contractors/visitors/patients
- All visitors to these premises should report to reception on
  arrival.
- A strict no-smoking policy applies to all users of our premises.
- No visitors will be allowed into areas other than the general
  waiting area, adjoining corridors and toilets unless accompanied
  by a member of staff.

A copy of this and all other practice policies will be issued to staff
on commencement of employment. Additional copies of each
practice policy will be in the Health and Safety manual located
at: _____ .

This and all policies will be reviewed annually and kept up to date
as the needs of the practice and legislation change.

Signed _____   Date _____

Manual handling

The most frequently given cause of a work-related back or limb problem by workers is manual handling (cited by 52% of those with a back problem), followed by posture (28%) and repetitive work (18%).[41,42] Incorrect handling of loads causes many injuries, resulting in pain, time off work and even permanent disablement.

The Manual Handling Regulations 1992 apply to all manual handling operations, including lifting, lowering, pushing, pulling, carrying, holding or moving loads, whether by hand or other bodily force. They cover the nature of the force applied, i.e. duration, frequency, magnitude and postures adopted, and apply to animate loads, such as moving patients, as well as inanimate.

It may be that 'lifting' is not an issue in your place of work, but it is worth remembering that if staff do not regularly use physical effort they are probably in a more vulnerable position if they are required to do so on an odd occasion than someone who handles heavy weights on a daily basis. One important mechanism for reducing strain on the lumbar spine is the pressure created within the abdomen by having strong abdominal muscles, which effectively splints the spine from the front.

Loads carried compress the intervertebral discs. This is not usually a problem if the natural curves of the spine are maintained. But if the back is bent forwards or sideways or twisted, an uneven stress is placed on one part of the disc or the ligaments around it, and damage may occur. Loads carried nearer the spine are easier to control and create less strain on the spine. Twisting, stooping or reaching upwards with a load places more strain on the spine, and the arms are also prone to injury. Loads which are awkward, bulky, prone to shift or have to be handled in limited spaces or with poor lighting, add to potential hazards. The age of staff, their fitness and whether they are, or have recently been, pregnant needs to be considered in assessing the risk of manual handling operations.

Because individuals' capabilities vary, there are no specific maximum weights which should not be exceeded when lifting objects. However, the table below gives some guidelines.

Type of lifting	Maximum weight	
	Male	Female
• lifted from below knee height or above shoulder height if close to the body	10 kg	7 kg
• if further away than the length of your forearm	5 kg	$3\frac{1}{2}$ kg
• lifting at waist height close to the body	25 kg	17 kg
• if lifting involves twisting weight reduced by 10–20%		

If the lifting is done repeatedly within a short time, reductions in weight must be made:

- by 20% if repeated once or twice per minute
- by up to 80% if repeated more than 12 times per minute.

Sometimes there are simple solutions to ergonomic problems, e.g. someone else holding a door open for a colleague carrying a bulky item, or using a handling strap to move a patient from a wheelchair to the toilet, or taking meal breaks in easy chairs, rather than using the same desk chair all day long.

There is some evidence that general fitness helps to maintain strength and flexibility and thus prevent back problems, and you should be able to advise staff and patients about the availability of local facilities.

Establishing a manual handling policy

Primary care is an obvious example of where staff are at risk with respect to manual handling. Take into account the task, the load, the working environment and the individual capabilities in determining what measures may be taken to minimise the risk of injury to people carrying out the operations.

There are four key steps to implementing a manual handling policy:

- avoid manual handling operations where reasonably practicable
- adequately assess any hazardous operations that cannot be avoided
- reduce the risk of injury as far as practicable
- re-evaluate your risks from manual handling for your workforce.

A model for a manual handling policy for general medical or pharmacy practice

Statement of policy
The practice has a commitment on lifting and handling to:

1 reduce manual handling of heavy loads where that is reasonably practicable
2 reduce the risk of back injury caused by the manual handling of heavy loads
3 provide appropriate training in suitable lifting and handling techniques.

It is the joint responsibility of the GP/pharmacist employer and the named staff member concerned to decide on the appropriate methods for lifting heavy loads and the employee's responsibility to:

1 take account of the weight involved and arrange help with lifting (from other people or equipment) where necessary
2 use the correct lifting technique at all times.

General arrangements
- Detailed information is available on safety procedures and techniques applicable to each area of the practice.
- Every member of staff who is required to carry out lifting and handling tasks as part of their normal duties will receive annual training in lifting and handling techniques.
- Risk assessment will be carried out in all areas of the practice to include non-patient and patient loads by . . . . (appointed 'competent person').
- Records will be kept of all non-patient load risk assessments for each area of the practice.
- Remedial action will be taken to negate any risks identified.

This policy will be kept up to date and reviewed annually.

Signed . . . . (GP/pharmacist employer)

Date . . . . Review date . . . .

Guidelines for lifting in unusual circumstances[43]

1 Patient with cardiac or respiratory arrest lying on the floor: continue resuscitation on the floor until the patient can be lifted onto sheet or equivalent and there are a minimum of four people to lift.

2 Unconscious patient lying on the floor: place the patient in the unconscious position on the floor until at least four people are available to lift.

3 A patient who has a fall in a confined space: slide the patient into a more spacious area; consider calling for an ambulance if suspected fracture.

Ergonomics and posture

Ergonomics focuses on the interaction between the worker and the job. The science of ergonomics seeks to improve the match between the job and the employee's physical ability and workload capacity – combining the elements of comfort, health and productivity. It is important to minimise the likelihood of causing back pain by looking at the posture people adopt during the working day and the strain put on the spine by incorrect handling of loads.

Good posture involves maintaining the spine and other joints in positions which create the least strain. The natural curves of the spine should be preserved, reducing disc compression and ligament strain, and other joints should be sufficiently well-positioned that strain on ligaments and tendons is minimised.

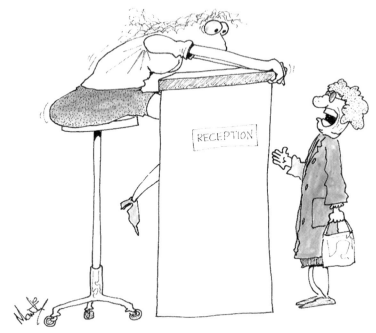

Postural strains on staff can present problems when they occur many times in a day, or for long periods. It is easy for someone to reach into a stretched position once in a while, but if staff are asked to do so for even quite a short period, strains can occur. So, while it may be no problem for you to bend down to knee height to collect a document emerging from a printer once, it could place an unreasonable strain on a receptionist's back if she were to do this continuously for 15 minutes.

Postural strains may include the kind of working position required because of the furniture used, but they may also be related to the pace of the work, the lack of rest periods and other psychological issues which impair the physical ability of the staff member, and can lead to work-related stress and musculoskeletal disorders.

Work with visual display unit (VDU) screen equipment and other similar equipment is not high-risk, but can lead to muscular and other physical problems, eye fatigue and mental stress. The Display Screen Equipment (DSE) Regulations 1992 aim to ensure that these problems are prevented by paying attention to the correct ergonomic set-up of the workstation, the working environment and the tasks performed. The regulations apply to all 'regular users' of display screen equipment, which could, therefore, cover most practice employees including the GP/pharmacist themselves.

The definition of a VDU 'user' includes anyone using a VDU for continuous periods of an hour or more on most days, who has to transfer information quickly to or from the screen, or anyone using a VDU more or less continuously on most days.

Employers are obliged to assess not only the VDU itself but the whole workstation, including seating, environmental factors, the software and task design. The VDU user can make the assessment himself or herself using a standard checklist, such as that in the HSE booklet *VDUs – an easy guide to the regulations.* (*See* Appendix 2.)

Consider what kinds of postural strain are placed on staff through: poorly designed furniture and equipment, poor arrangement of work and equipment, prolonged activity and stress. Physical factors in the practice environment causing ergonomic problems include:

- frequent repetitive movements on a keyboard
- awkward posture at a reception desk or counter
- lifting
- seating – relative to workstation
- posture sitting or standing
- VDUs
- standing
- lack of rest facilities.

Personal safety

The problem of aggression and violence at work is common in the general working population, with around 35 000 people in the UK being attacked at work each year. The British Crime Survey reported that health professionals appear to be at higher risk of work-related violence (including woundings, common assault, robbery and snatch theft) than the general population, with records showing a frequency of 580 incidents per 10 000 nurses and midwives in 1995.[44]

Nurses are particularly vulnerable to aggression and violence: some have a great deal of daily one-to-one contact with patients who are mentally ill or disturbed, in circumstances where emotions run high and patients or relatives can suddenly become irrational or aggressive. Nurses, doctors and pharmacists who visit patients in their own homes are often unaware of danger, because their caring nature and their role as the patients' advocate makes them relatively unsuspicious.

Preventing an episode of aggression and violence from occurring in the first place will include:[35]

- avoiding potentially dangerous situations, especially when on visits to patients' homes
- learning how to defuse tense confrontations
- improving the workplace organisation so that the service provided is efficient
- devising a workplace policy to handle a violent or aggressive incident
- equipping staff with assertiveness and anger-management skills
- offering support to staff who have been victims of attack or abuse
- learning from any violent episode and making changes to avoid a recurrence
- reporting the incident to the police, to prevent a recurrence.

Verbal abuse is at one end of a continuous spectrum that ends in physical assault. Such episodes should be treated seriously and not dismissed as trivial just because they were not accompanied by physical attack.

The law on health and safety at work applies to risks from violence, just as it does to other risks at work. The practice, as an employer, needs to recognise the importance of staff feeling safe and supported. Some patients and their relatives, as well as members of the public, may pose a risk to GPs and staff within the isolation of a home or practice setting. This includes the vulnerability of staff travelling alone in cars, especially during the hours of darkness. Working alone increases certain types of risk to staff and requires separate assessment.

Everyone in the general medical or pharmacy practice should be familiar with a workplace policy to reduce the likelihood of aggression and violence flaring at work, to defuse any such incident effectively, to summon help as necessary, and to counsel and support any victim afterwards.

The practice must ensure that appropriate training, guidance and other relevant support/equipment is available to staff to minimise such risks as identified. A written policy will show the practice commitment to providing safe working conditions for staff.

The policy should include:

- a statement of intent to protect staff from work-related violence
- a definition of violence and aggression that covers non-physical as well as physical violence and aggression, from other members of staff, patients, relatives and members of the public
- legal obligations
- specific roles and responsibilities of staff and management
- measures to reduce the risks of violence and aggression in everyday working procedures and emergency situations
- provision of staff training
- provision of reporting and recording incidents
- provision of post-trauma support.

A model for a personal safety policy

Statement of policy
The practice has a commitment to:

1 protect the health and safety of staff at work
2 protect the health and safety of others who might be affected by the way they go about their work.

The practice will take all practicable steps to:

1 assess risks to personal safety of employees (including risk of criminal attack)
2 identify the precautions needed
3 provide arrangements for the effective management of precautions
4 appoint competent personnel to oversee or advise on personal safety
5 provide information and training to employees to minimise the risk to their personal safety.

Overall responsibility for personal safety: . . . .
(GP/pharmacist)

Management and implementation of the policy: . . . .
(appointed 'competent person')

Responsibility for training in personal safety: . . . .

Employees' responsibilities:

1   to take reasonable care of the health and safety of him/herself
    and other people
2   to report incidents of violence, aggression and accidents.

Accident Recording Book sited: . . . .

This policy will be kept up to date and reviewed annually.

Signed . . . .   (GP/pharmacist employer or deputy)

Date   Review date . . . .

Accident reporting and Reporting of Injuries, Diseases and Dangerous Occurrence Regulations (RIDDOR), 1995

The practice internal reporting, recording and investigation systems need to capture information about all accidents, including those that are of a less serious nature. All accidents and near misses (incidents), whether producing injury or not, must be reported verbally or in writing within the practice. Careful reporting of any accidents or incidents should identify potential problems and prompt remedial action, helping the practice to monitor the effectiveness of the precautions taken.

All practices should have a system for the reporting and investigation of accidents and injuries in the workplace to comply with RIDDOR, which requires employers to report and keep records of serious accidents to, and violent assaults on, employees. Injuries, diseases and occurrences in specified categories should be notified to the environmental health department of the local authority. Failure to comply is a criminal offence (Accident Reporting Regulations).

The duty of notification is on the employer. A fatal or major injury to anyone sustained in an accident connected with your practice or pharmacy business should be immediately notified by telephone to the HSE. Reporting should otherwise be by post, using standard forms

(F2508 for injuries and dangerous occurrences, F2508A for occupational diseases) available from HSE Books. Report any injury to a general practice or pharmacy staff member who falls at work or injures themselves in other ways (perhaps lifting a patient) and subsequently takes more than three days off work or is unable to do their normal work for more than three days. There are other illnesses relevant to a primary care setting that should be notified that are outside the scope of

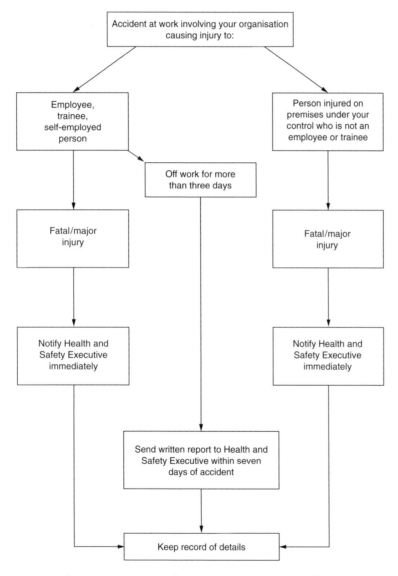

Figure 5.1: Guide to Reporting of Injuries, Diseases and Dangerous Occurrence Regulations (RIDDOR), 1995.

this text on back pain and back problems (*see* Appendix 2 for further reading).

Figure 5.1 shows the reporting procedures for informing the Health and Safety Executive of more serious accidents.

A good accident/incident reporting system will have the following characteristics:

1 An accident should be reported as soon as possible to an appropriate person.
2 Details of any accidents or injuries should be recorded in an accident book, including the:
   – date, time and nature of the incident/accident
   – name and full occupation of employee
   – place where the incident occurred
   – description of the circumstances.
3 If the accident is significant, practice insurers may need to be informed. It is essential to keep and make available detailed information in the event of legal action being taken.
4 Report accidents and occurrences specified by the regulations on form F2508 (or F2508A for specific diseases) available from the HSE.
5 The accident should be investigated and action taken to prevent recurrence – noting the events that led up to the accident and the cause of the accident.

Disability Discrimination Act (DDA) 1995

Disability is defined as: 'a physical or mental impairment which has a substantial and long-term adverse effect on a person's ability to carry out normal day-to-day activities.' The Act covers people with a past disability as well as a present one.[45]

Long-term effects include those that have lasted or are likely to last 12 months or more, whether continuously or by periodic recurrence. Normal day-to-day activities cover the following broad categories:

- mobility
- manual dexterity
- physical co-ordination
- continence
- ability to lift, carry or move ordinary objects
- speech, hearing or eyesight
- memory, or ability to concentrate, learn or understand
- being able to recognise physical dangers.

The Act places obligations on employers with businesses that employ 15 or more employees. But the principles of the Act are good employment practice and should therefore be followed irrespective of practice size. The Act makes it unlawful for employers to discriminate against current or prospective employees with disabilities on account of their disability.

Employers must make reasonable changes to premises, work practices and employment arrangements, e.g. hours of work and work breaks, to accommodate a disabled employee.

So, a GP/pharmacist or practice manager should be aware of the provisions of the DDA if a member of staff is, or becomes, disabled by back pain or back problems.

Reflection exercises

Exercise 13 (for GP and pharmacy employers and practice managers). Monitoring compliance with health and safety legislation

Please tick relevant boxes.

1 Has the practice written policies for managing the following issues?

	Yes	No	Don't know
(a) health and safety	☐	☐	☐
(b) manual handling	☐	☐	☐
(c) working environment	☐	☐	☐
(d) personal safety	☐	☐	☐

2 Responsibility for formulating policies within the practice is with:

	Yes	No	Don't know
GP/pharmacist	☐	☐	☐
practice manager	☐	☐	☐
staff member	☐	☐	☐
other:			

3 Are the written policies listed as existing in question 1 above readily to hand?

readily to hand	☐
some are to hand, but not others	☐
could be found if responsible person searched for them	☐
goodness knows where they are	☐

4   There is a named person responsible for:

	Yes	No	Don't know
reviewing and acting on policies	☐	☐	☐
first aid and maintaining first aid stock annually	☐	☐	☐

5   Risk assessments according to Health and Safety legislation are carried out:

annually in every area of the practice   ☐
at least annually in a few areas of the practice   ☐
carried out only following an incident   ☐
risk assessments are not done at all   ☐

6   All accidents (however trivial) are recorded by means of an accident book:

always   ☐
sometimes   ☐
never   ☐
don't know   ☐

7   The information collected about types of accidents/injuries concerns:

slips, trips or falls   ☐
manual handling – patient   ☐
manual handling – non-patient   ☐
struck by moving machine, vehicle or object   ☐
assault   ☐
working environment   ☐
other   ☐

8   Recorded information about accidents is used to make changes and avoid future accidents:

always   ☐
sometimes   ☐
never   ☐
don't know   ☐

9   The following are available to staff in the practice/pharmacy:

pre-employment screening   ☐
induction in health and safety information   ☐
health and safety training   ☐
health surveillance where appropriate   ☐
information on health and safety matters   ☐

10 Staff who have received training on the prevention of back pain in
    last three years are:
    GP/pharmacist ☐
    practice manager ☐
    counter staff/reception/clerical staff ☐
    practice nurses ☐
    cleaners/domestic staff ☐

Conclude: what changes will you make as a result of carrying out this
exercise?

Exercise 14 (for GP and pharmacy employers and practice managers). Review your safety and security arrangements to prevent the likelihood of violence and aggression occurring to staff in your workplace

How does your workplace or organisation measure up? Circle the types
of systems or procedures that exist:

Preventive	*In response to a violent episode*
Staff training	Support staff
Team approach	Report episode
Adequate staffing	Analyse incident
Secure premises	Discuss changes and solutions
Surgery alarms	Change systems or procedures
Good environment	Review policy
Good communication	Prosecute perpetrators of violence
Practice policy	Make structural changes to
Planned interventions for different	increase security
eventualities	
General awareness of danger	
Good organisation	
Culture of concern for staff	

What are the most dangerous situations **for you** at work and what
changes can you make to minimise the chances of aggression and
violence arising?

Potentially threatening situations   Intended changes

-
-
-

Exercise 15 (for GPs, community nurses, therapists, pharmacists and staff)

Look at the illustrations, which show rather disorganised practice and pharmacy workplaces that are jam-packed full of hazards. Try to spot the hazards in both – they are different and depict hazards not specific to medical or pharmacy premises but which might be found in any workplace. Most of these hazards could cause back pain from staff tripping, lifting, carrying loads, adopting poor posture, etc.

(i) Spot the hazards in the fictitious general practice premises

Try to find at least 20 hazards. Think of all kinds of hazards and not just those directly related to causing back pain. Then check against our answers.

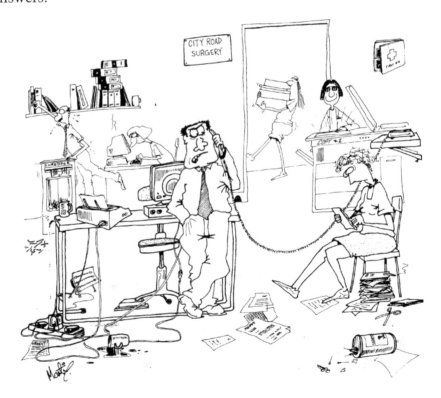

Spot the hazards in the fictitious general practice premises – we've found 30:

- Sharps box on floor spilling out needles
- Coffee cup spilling its contents on the floor
- Coffee mug by printer has been repaired, so is dangerous
- Trailing wires from the phone and computer and printer
- Overloaded adapter with many wires plugged into the socket
- Open electric fire without guard
- Electric fire is near to trailing lead
- Unattended cigarette butt burning on table
- Secretary's cigarette lying on top of pile of papers by her chair
- Scissors lying open on floor
- Electric lead to computer frayed in the middle
- Computer chair propped up on books, as a wheel is missing
- Printer almost falling off edge of table
- Urgent notice lying on floor
- Private letter lying on floor
- Secretary sitting just below telephone shelf, likely to hit head when she gets up
- Poor posture of secretary
- Poor posture of computer operator in background
- Dangerous pile of files on shelf might fall off onto person below or create new hazard on floor
- Coffee mug poised on high shelf above computer operator – hot contents might tip over her
- Man over-reaching for books on high shelf
- Man in background poorly balanced and in danger of catching fingers and tie in the shredder
- Shredder has spilt waste paper on the floor – fire hazard
- Letters on floor by secretary are fire hazard
- Papers and letters on floor create potential hazard which might trip up passer-by
- Woman in background carrying awkward and heavy load
- Photocopier lid open, causing possible eye strain hazard to operator
- First aid box has open door
- Mouse hole – there may be vermin
- Overcrowded room – threatens privacy of confidential phonecalls

(ii) Spot the hazards in the fictitious pharmacy premises

Try to find at least 20 hazards. Think of all kinds of hazards and not just those directly related to causing back pain. Then check against our answers.

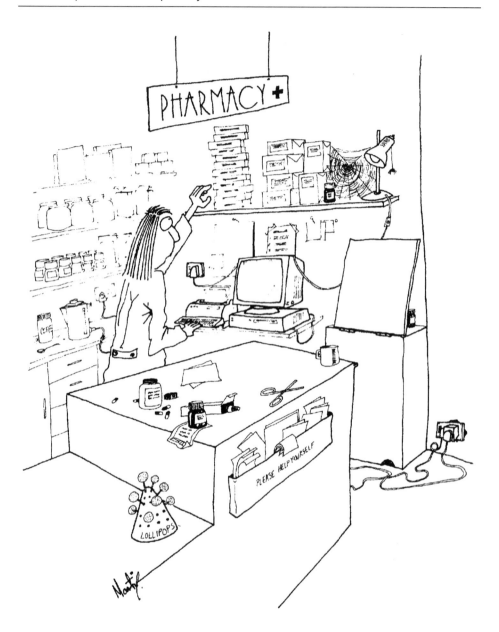

Spot the hazards in the fictitious pharmacy premises – we've found 22:

- Trailing leads on floor
- Trailing lead to desk lamp, perched dangerously on shelf
- Adaptor in socket appears to be overloaded
- Kettle lead trailing
- Unhygienic refreshment area not separated from where medicines are prepared
- Dangerous stacks on shelf
- Notice 'please help yourself' by bottle of tablets/tube of medication
- Loose tablets on counter by open bottle
- Prescription lying under tablet bottle – might be lost or stolen. Breach of confidentiality if customers can read it
- Selling lollipops next to tablets – might encourage children to regard tablets as sweets
- Scissors open on counter near to lollipops
- Coffee mug on edge of counter – danger of spillage to staff and customers
- Counter flap left up, potential danger of it dropping down on to someone's fingers, allowing public easy access to dispensary stores or leaving pharmacist vulnerable to attack
- Tablet bottle out of sight behind flap
- Notices haphazardly stuck on wall – they could be important, and fall off
- Spider and cobwebs – the place hasn't been cleaned properly
- Mouse hole – may be vermin
- Pharmacist reaching for items loosely stacked above head height likely to trigger cascade of items
- Used coffee spoon lying around dispensary
- General disorganisation and chaos
- No chair at workstation so pharmacist has to stand
- Keyboard sited awkwardly in relation to the computer screen

Exercise 16 (for GP and pharmacy employers, community nurses, therapists and members of practice or pharmacy staff). Undertake a risk assessment of your workplace

The following risk assessment check list incorporates assessment of general health and safety, manual handling, ergonomics and posture, accidents and injuries.

Hazard

Access to premises:

paths
illumination
steps
doorways

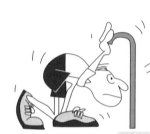

- Maintenance of uneven paths
- Security lights
- Ramps
- Door width for wheelchair access

Floors/stairs:

surfaces – worn carpet
wet/slippery
obstructions
illumination

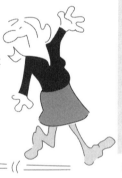

- Replace floor coverings/ stick down loose edges
- Make sure toys do not present a risk to users of the premises
- Ensure that goods delivered are placed where they will not cause an obstruction
- See that there is adequate lighting, especially in stairways

Reception/counter area:

height of counter
seating
telephone
windows
position of equipment

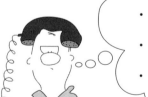

- Is counter suitable height for all staff – is a step needed for shorter staff if standing for long periods?
- Are chairs adjustable, and with lumbar support?
- Do staff hold the phone by bending their neck sideways? Would headphones help?
- Are windows stiff; are curtains easily accessible, or are steps needed?
- Is office equipment arranged to reduce twisting or bending?

DATE . . . .

Is there a hazard from the task, the load, the working environment, the capability of the staff?	How can this be avoided or minimised?	Is the risk adequately controlled? Yes/No	Further action needed

Hazard

Filing/storage area:

height and arrangement of shelves

- Does the filing system require staff to twist in order to see the names?
- Could rotating files or forward-facing cabinets be used instead?
- Are shelves too high for the safe lifting of storage boxes? Either split up the contents into smaller parts which can be lifted safely, or use only shelves at a safe height

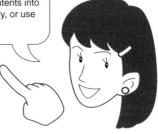

Using the computer:

chair
footrest
keyboard
screen
lighting
variation in tasks

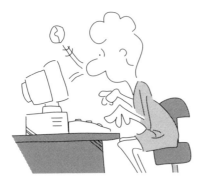

- Adjustable height of seat and backrest on chair
- Footrest available
- Space around keyboard for wrist support, forearms are horizontal
- Document-holder positioned to minimise neck strain
- Screen adjustable at optimum height (eyes level with top of screen, viewing display by looking at a slightly downwards angle)
- No glare, brightness adjusted for clear visibility
- Other equipment used should be easily accessible without straining (e.g. printer)
- Make sure there are no trailing cables
- Work should allow frequent breaks or change in tasks to minimise strain

Consultation/treatment room in medical practice:

examination couch

Couch height should be adjustable, or step available for patients

DATE . . . .

Is there a hazard from the task, the load, the working environment, the capability of the staff?	How can this be avoided or minimised?	Is the risk adequately controlled? Yes/No	Further action needed

Hazard

Working outside the practice/transporting yourself and your equipment:

lifting equipment into a car
positioning equipment in patient's home

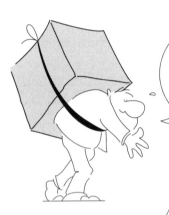

- Avoid stooping while lifting
- Train staff in manual handling
- Where possible, use light equipment
- Assess carefully heavy loads such as oxygen cylinders, which may require a specialist trolley/vehicle hoist

Maintenance staff:

vacuum cleaner
staff's physical fitness
wheelie bin
buckets
large containers of
    supplies
moving furniture
changing light bulbs

- Consider lighter vacuum cleaner or additional cleaner for use upstairs
- Provide sack truck for heavy stock
- Pre-employment screening and manual handling training for all staff
- Fill buckets, pouring several smaller quantities into bucket on floor; don't lift heavy bucket out of sink
- Ensure sufficient staff to help each other with awkward loads or jobs, e.g. changing fluorescent tubes, which may need two sets of steps

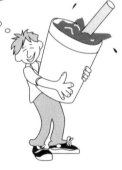

Moving patients in the practice/patient's home:

from chair to
    standing
from standing to
    lying on a bed
from wheelchair to
    toilet
collapsed on floor
    to sitting

- Manual handling training for all staff
- Sufficient staff available
- Hoist available if necessary
- Use adjustable bed/couch
- Provide toilet in surgery large enough for wheelchair access

DATE . . . .

Is there a hazard from the task, the load, the working environment, the capability of the staff?	How can this be avoided or minimised?	Is the risk adequately controlled? Yes/No	Further action needed

Hazard

Working in the community:

vulnerable staff
difficult working environment

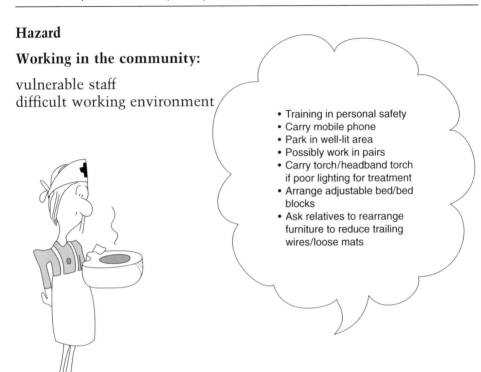

- Training in personal safety
- Carry mobile phone
- Park in well-lit area
- Possibly work in pairs
- Carry torch/headband torch if poor lighting for treatment
- Arrange adjustable bed/bed blocks
- Ask relatives to rearrange furniture to reduce trailing wires/loose mats

Conclusion to risk assessment exercise:

1 What hazards have you identified?
2 Do you and others in your practice team know how to avoid, minimise or eliminate those hazards? If not, include these topics in your PDP or practice-based learning plan.
3 What is your action plan for your risk reduction programme? Be specific – give objectives, method, expected outcomes, timetable.

Now that you have completed one or more of the interactive reflection exercises in this chapter, transfer the information from this needs assessment to the empty template of the personal development plan on pages 107–110 if you are working on your own learning plan; or to the practice personal and professional development plan on pages 133–136 if you are working on a practice-team learning plan – if this risk assessment is appropriate to the topic you are focusing on. The conclusions made at the end of each exercise will feature in the action plan. Don't forget to keep evidence of your learning in your personal portfolio.

DATE . . . .

Is there a hazard from the task, the load, the working environment, the capability of the staff?	How can this be avoided or minimised?	Is the risk adequately controlled? Yes/No	Further action needed

Draw up and apply your personal development plan focusing on the clinical management of low back pain

You will probably be interested in making the effective clinical management of back pain a focus of your personal development plan (PDP) if you are a GP or therapist providing care to patients, a community nurse advising patients, or a pharmacist supporting GPs and advising customers with back pain.

- Read through Worked example 1 on pages 111–118 of how a **GP** might draw up a PDP focused around the clinical management of back pain.
- Read through Worked example 2 on pages 119–124 of how a **pharmacist** might draw up a PDP focused around giving reliable advice to customers with back pain or back problems.
- Read through Worked example 3 on pages 125–130 of how a **nurse** might draw up a PDP focused around her or his own back care. Any health professional might generalise from this plan to their own situation – it is not specific to nurses.

The examples given are very comprehensive and you may not want to include so much in your own PDP. You might include different topics and educational activities because your needs and circumstances are different from the example practitioners here.

Transfer the information about your learning needs from the reflection exercises at the end of the chapters you have completed so far to the empty template of the PDP that follows.

Look at what you have recorded – for instance:

- Do you have a practice protocol?
- Do you monitor that protocol?

- Do you comply with best practice in diagnosing, advising, investigating and treating patients?
- Do you know to whom to refer people with back pain – and when and where?

The conclusions you have made at the end of each exercise will feature in the action plan of your PDP. Some more ideas about the preliminary information you should be gathering for your PDP are given in the boxes of the template.

It might take around ten hours to draw up your learning plan, depending on what you do in the way of the preliminary needs assessment, and the extent of learning and changes you undertake. The reflective exercises at the end of each chapter will fulfil most of your needs assessment – the time taken will depend on whether you undertake all the exercises or delegate them to a member of staff, or whether you are already performing well in these exercises. Incorporate learning about other important priority areas into your annual plan, too, such as cancer, coronary heart disease, diabetes, etc.

Template for your personal development plan

Photocopy the four pages if you want to use the chart again for other topics

---

What topic(s)?

Justify why topic(s) is/are a priority:
a personal priority?
a practice and professional priority?
a district or national priority?

(It may be a critical incident, or new guidelines that you mention here)

| Exercise 3 |

Who else will be included in your personal development plan?
(Any colleagues share your interest?)

| Exercise 7 |

What baseline information will you collect?
(See reflective exercises at ends of each chapter, e.g. the existence or absence of a clinical protocol; extent to which you adhere to best practice, etc.)

| Selection of Exercises 1–16 |

What are your learning needs and how do they match those of the practice?
(Weigh the strategic or business needs of the practice and your needs here)

Patient or public input to your plan
(You might ask patients to comment on your current performance or the resources available, e.g. for investigation or referral)

How will you prioritise your learning needs?
(Are some learning needs more significant than others; are resources available?)

Objectives of your PDP arising from the preliminary data-gathering exercise
(So what exactly do you intend to achieve from your learning?)

How you might integrate the 14 components of clinical governance[3] into your PDP, focusing on the clinical management of back pain
Transfer the clinical governance checklist that you completed in Exercise 1 at the end of Chapter 1 here (*see* pages 13–15).

Establishing a learning culture:

Managing resources and services:

Establishing a research and development culture:

Reliable and accurate data:

Evidence-based practice and policy:

Confidentiality:

Health gain:

Coherent team:

Audit and evaluation:

Meaningful involvement of patients and the public:

Health promotion:

Risk management:

Accountability and performance:

Core requirements:

What additional resources will you require to execute your plan and from where do you hope to obtain them?

How much protected time will you have to undertake the learning described in your plan?

Action plan (include objectives, timetabled action, expected outcomes)
(Be specific. Draw on your conclusions that followed the reflection exercises. Be realistic about what you can achieve. Define outcomes now so that you can review what you have set out to achieve at a later date and know whether you have been successful and what else you should be planning to do.)

How will you evaluate your learning plan?
(Who will be responsible for what?)

How will you know when you have achieved your objectives?
(How will you measure success?)

How will you disseminate the learning from your plan and sustain the developments and new-found knowledge or skills?

How will you handle new learning requirements as they crop up?

Record of your learning about 'clinical management of back pain'
Write in topic, date, time spent, type of learning

	Activity 1	Activity 2	Activity 3	Activity 4
In-house formal learning				
External courses				
Informal and personal				
Qualifications and/or experience gained				

Worked example 1: a personal development plan for a GP focusing on the clinical management of back pain

What topic? Clinical management of back pain

Justify why topic is a priority:

(i) *a practice and professional priority?* Unnecessary X-rays expose patients to avoidable risks from radiation. Back pain may be reduced if GPs recommend patients take exercise and continue normal activities rather than resting.

(ii) *a district priority?* Limiting the numbers of inappropriate back X-rays should reduce costs and preventable ill health.

(iii) *a national priority?* Appropriate early management of acute back pain should reduce the development of long-term chronic back pain and sickness absence.

Who will be included in your personal development plan?

You might work on your own or liaise with a:

- GP
- practice nurse
- practice manager
- community pharmacist
- community physiotherapist
- osteopath
- chiropodist/podiatrist
- chiropractor
- patient.

Where are you now – baseline information?

You might ask the local X-ray department to supply quarterly data of your referrals. A baseline audit by one of the receptionists might look at how often 'occupation' was recorded in patients' records for those suffering from back pain. You might keep a log of patients consulting with back pain and note down how often they are advised about exercise or the possible benefits of alternative therapies.

You might include:

- whether your practice has a protocol or guidelines for best practice in managing back pain or problems or not. If not, describe your usual practice for patients with differing degrees of back pain, over time
- whether you know about the range of practitioners providing alternative medicine and where to refer patients – such as osteopaths, herbalists, aromatherapists, acupuncturists, chiropractors, homoeopaths or remedial therapists. Are you familiar with their qualifications, the range of therapies, the evidence in support of the alternative therapies, availability and cost etc.?
- audits of aspects of clinical management: for example, numbers of patients prescribed anti-inflammatory drugs for back pain, number X-rayed, numbers receiving magnetic resonance scans (MRI), numbers referred to NHS physiotherapy and for orthopaedic opinions from hospital consultants. You might compare your clinical management with that of other GPs
- extent to which you promote exercise for all patients, especially those with back problems. Is there an exercise referral scheme to local leisure centres? Is it used? Do you know what sport and leisure services are available locally – swimming pools, gyms, sports or walking clubs, etc?

What information will you obtain about your learning needs?

You could undertake a significant event audit after a patient who was on anti-inflammatory drugs for back pain had a sudden fatal haematemesis. A district-wide audit of the numbers of X-ray investigations of the lumbar–sacral spine might reveal whether you/your practice make comparatively more or less referrals than other similar practices.

You could undertake an audit of the next 20 consecutive patients who have had back pain for at least three months to see how their experiences tally with how you expect your services to operate. You might find that there was a reason why they did not access your care before, if this is their first visit. You may find that they have not been advised to stay active or that they ignored such advice and went to bed (this might reveal learning needs – not being able to convince the patients of recommended practice).

How do your learning needs match those of the practice as a whole?

You could draw up a protocol or guidelines for the practice, based on recommended best practice in back care management; or adopt recommendations from elsewhere. If current practice is demonstrated to be putting patients at unnecessary risk by over-investigation with X-rays, giving inappropriate medication, or costing the patients avoidable time off work, then everyone should agree to adhere to the protocols, even if not particularly eager to learn more themselves about managing back pain.

Patient or public input to your plan

You might hold an open evening to which practice staff contribute short talks or demonstrations of best practice in back care. A physiotherapist or osteopath might show people how to lift heavy objects, do back-strengthening exercises and maintain good posture; a spokesman from leisure services might describe their equipment; a GP or chiropractor might talk about what people with back pain can do for themselves; a podiatrist might stress the importance of good footwear to correct an abnormal gait.

You might ask patients with back pain to tell you how you might improve your services. For instance, it may be that a back support is available at reception if those with back problems have a long wait to see the doctor and want to ease the discomfort of sitting on the surgery chairs; or that you need simpler and clearer patient literature.

How will you prioritise your learning needs?

You only have a limited time to spend, so try to focus on issues on which to improve, so that there are maximum benefits for patient care.

Aims of the personal development plan arising from the preliminary data-gathering exercise

To meet the objectives of the *Back in Work* initiative:[46]

- 'to reduce the misery and cost of back pain to those in the workplace' for patients in general.
- to 'promote good practice in back care management within a framework that includes prevention, assessment, treatment and rehabilitation'.

How you might integrate the 14 components of clinical governance into your personal development plan focusing on 'back pain'

Establishing a learning culture: you might use your interest in back pain and what you find out about practice performance to set up a practice meeting and feed the information back to the rest of the practice.

Managing resources and services: referring to a physiotherapist earlier might reduce chronic back pain; linking to a leisure centre might reduce NHS costs in the long term.

Establishing a research and development culture: incorporating research recommendations into everyday practice (e.g. that exercise and normal daily activities shorten the length of the episode) demonstrates how research can be applied in practice to make an impact on the quality of patient care.

Reliable and accurate data: collect information about cases of back pain seen (numbers, location, severity, length of episode, referrals etc.) and monitor adherence to practice protocols, such as appropriate referrals for X-rays.

Evidence-based practice and policy: knowing the evidence for all types of therapies from conventional NHS care to a range of alternative therapies will help you to explain the options to patients in an informed way.

Confidentiality: the consulting patient should feel that information from his or her medical records will be shared on a need-to-know basis with other health professionals. In any audit or research study, access to patients' medical records should be controlled and limited, with informed consent from the patients concerned and ethical approval of the study protocol if necessary.

Health gain: reduction in numbers of inappropriate X-rays will lessen the risk of adverse effects from unnecessary exposure to radiation. Early and effective interventions will get people back to normal activities as soon as possible.

Coherent team: more understanding of the roles and capabilities of therapists should result in a more coherent plan of management and more effective teamwork.

Audit and evaluation: audit any aspect of management, such as numbers and timing of referrals, promotion of normal activities and non-compliance, and make recommendations for evidence-based practice.

Meaningful involvement of patients and the public: consult people in your patient population with and without back problems about which alternative therapies should be available as part of the NHS.

Health promotion: exercise promotion is a mainstay of management.

Risk management: good risk management includes knowing the 'red flags' and 'yellow flags' to look out for which indicate serious spinal pathology or the potential for the condition to become chronic.

Accountability and performance: more teamworking will require everyone being clear about their roles and responsibilities in back pain management.

Core requirements: adherence to current recommended best practice should be cost-effective, with savings from reduction in inappropriate referrals for investigations, less time off work, earlier interventions by therapists.

Action plan

Agree who is involved/setting: as staff set out previously – specify names, posts.

Timetabled action:

start date:
by 3 months: preliminary data gathering and baseline of providers completed:

- is there a protocol for managing patients with mild, moderate and severe, acute and chronic back pain?
- numbers of staff; map expertise; list other providers
- referral patterns to X-ray, orthopaedic consultant, physiotherapy; prescribing patterns
- information about characteristics of those recorded on practice computer as having experienced back pain
- any relevant local and national priorities; and any additional associated resources that might be applied for?

by 4 months: review current performance:

- level of knowledge and use of practice protocol or guide for managing back problems; extent to which protocol or guide fits with best practice or others' back care management plans (e.g. hospital trust)
- audit of actual performance via pre-agreed criteria, e.g. with respect to referrals, promotion of exercise and normal activities
- compare performance with any or several of the 14 components of clinical governance, for example *risk management*.

by 6 months: identify solutions and associated training needs – plan learning activities and complete ongoing record of learning undertaken (*see* page 118):

- set up new systems for appropriate referral and management
- revise the practice protocol on the management of back problems/ pain as a practice team, with input from physiotherapist, to address identified gaps in care, having undertaken search for other evidence-based protocols. Agree roles and responsibilities as a team for delivering care and services according to protocol; certain staff attend external courses. Community pharmacist, health promotion facilitator and physiotherapist provide some in-house training to GPs and nurses.

by 12 months: make changes:

- clinicians adhere to practice protocol – as shown by repeat audit of increased/decreased referrals to X-ray, therapist, orthopaedic consultant as appropriate
- patients who are chronic back-pain sufferers take more exercise and pursue normal activities.

Expected outcomes: more effective management of back pain; better patient compliance with exercise and attendance at referrals; less sickness absence due to back pain.

What additional resources will you require?

You may need funds for a patient information leaflet carrying the most up-to-date advice.

Changes in referral patterns are likely as a result of learning activities – to reduce referral activity or divert referrals to less 'expensive' providers such as physiotherapists rather than orthopaedic consultants.

How much protected time will you allocate to undertaking the learning described in your plan?

That will depend on your circumstances, aspirations and needs.

How will you evaluate your learning plan?

You might re-audit any of the aspects of care and services that have featured so far.

How will you know when you have achieved your objectives?

Use the audit and survey methods described above and measure deviation from the agreed practice protocol.

Compare numbers of patients referred for exercise promotion, physiotherapy and X-ray investigation at baseline with those rates 12 months later.

How will you disseminate the learning from the plan to the rest of the practice team and patients? How will you sustain the new knowledge and skills?

You might write about it in a practice newsletter. Let all the staff know at practice meetings what progress has been made. You might want to talk about your provision at a community group meeting or at a neighbourhood forum. You might want to describe your success at a PCG/T meeting.

Pass on your skills and knowledge to others as required, review your protocol at set intervals to incorporate new information.

How will you handle new learning requirements as they crop up?

Undertake an audit of the next significant event to find out whether the preceding care and services adhered to the practice protocol. If not, determine why not; and if so, what else should be changed or learnt?

Record of your personal learning about 'back pain'

You would add the date, length of time spent etc. on each learning activity

	Activity 1: becoming familiar with other providers who might help prevent or treat back pain	Activity 2: best practice in the management of back pain	Activity 3: update on medication relevant to back pain
In-house formal learning	Physiotherapist, osteopath or chiropractor ran session for GPs, pharmacist nurses and non-clinical staff in local practice	Local radiologist, pharmacist, orthopaedic consultant, community physiotherapist contributed to 'roadshow' held in practice for patients and staff	Pharmacist updated GPs at in-practice lunchtime session; pharmacist swotted up the latest recommendations about medication and side effects prior to giving update
External courses	GP and pharmacist attended update seminar on back pain that included review of what other health professionals can do	GPs attended lunchtime lecture about best practice in the management of back pain	
Informal and personal	Practice staff pool literature mapping out complementary therapists – from Yellow Pages, unsolicited literature, health promotion – over coffee. Practice manager prints off list	GPs chatted with staff and practice manager in the course of the week about advantages of introducing an exercise prescription referral scheme. GPs swopped tips with other GPs at lunchtime lecture	Discussed results of audit of anti-inflammatory drugs as practice team at next meeting
Qualifications and/or experience gained	Certificate of attendance from course	GP registered for medical acupuncture course to extend range of treatments the practice can offer	Audits included in personal portfolio

Worked example 2: a personal development plan for a pharmacist focusing on back pain

What topic? Back pain: in relation to customers consulting with back pain.

Who chose topic? A pharmacist might choose to update their management of back pain if she or he realises that they are unsure of what best practice is, or what symptoms and signs indicate that referral to the GP or a therapist is appropriate, for instance.

Justify why topic is a priority:

(i) *a practice and professional priority?* Back pain may be reduced if pharmacists recommend patients and customers to take exercise and continue normal activities rather than resting.

(ii) *a district or national priority?* Appropriate early management of acute back pain will reduce the development of long-term chronic back pain.

Who will be included in your personal development plan?

You might work on your own or liaise with a:

- GP
- community physiotherapist
- osteopath
- chiropractor.

Where are you now – baseline information?

This might include:

- whether you have a protocol for best practice in advising about managing back pain
- whether you know of providers of alternative medicine and refer patients to them – such as osteopaths, herbalists, aromatherapists, acupuncturists, chiropractors, homoeopaths or remedial therapists – and are familiar with their qualifications, the range of therapies, the evidence in support of the alternative therapies, availability and cost etc.
- audits of your work in respect of advice about self-care, medication as described

- whether you and your pharmacy staff promote exercise for all patients, especially those with back problems. Is there an exercise referral scheme to local leisure centres? Is it used? Do you know what leisure services are available locally?

What information will you obtain about your individual learning needs?

You may undertake a significant event audit after a patient who was on anti-inflammatory drugs for back pain has a sudden fatal haematemesis.

Think how often you receive feedback from local GP practices about particular patient events. Could you encourage this?

You could undertake an audit of the next 20 consecutive patients who have had back pain (e.g. Exercise 6).

How do your learning needs match those of the pharmacy practice as a whole?

You may find that the learning needs of your pharmacy staff are similar to your own in respect of non-clinical advice to help those with back pain, such as location of leisure and sports facilities, whereabouts and nature of complementary therapists, etc.

Patient or public input to your plan

As a pharmacist you might ask patients with back pain to tell you how you might improve your services. For instance, they might suggest that you need simpler and clearer patient literature.

How will you prioritise your learning needs?

You only have a limited time to spend, so try to focus on issues where there are potentially the greatest benefits for patient care.

Aims of the PDP arising from the preliminary data-gathering exercise

To meet the objectives of the *Back in Work* initiative:[46]

- 'to reduce the misery and cost of back pain to those in the workplace' for patients in general
- to 'promote good practice in back care management within a framework that includes prevention, assessment, treatment and rehabilitation'.

How you might integrate the 14 components of clinical governance into your PDP focusing on back pain

Establishing a learning culture: teach your counter staff about advising customers with back pain appropriately.

Managing resources and services: have an easily accessible catalogue of aids, such as physical back supports.

Establishing a research and development culture: share the evidence for best practice in back care with staff, discussing how to apply that in your own workplace for customers and staff. This might concern exercise promotion, medication, complementary therapies.

Reliable and accurate data: keep accurate records to be able to advise customers and minimise drug interactions from prescribed and OTC drugs.

Evidence-based practice and policy: base pharmacy practices and your advice on the evidence.

Confidentiality: offer opportunities for customers to be able to talk privately with the pharmacist or counter staff.

Health gain: minimise customers' exposure to potentially harmful drugs such as NSAIDs when they can be avoided.

Coherent team: you, the counter and dispensary staff should all be clear about your roles and responsibilities and how each person fits within the team.

Audit and evaluation: undertake systematic audit of advice given.

Meaningful involvement of customers and the general public: ask customers about opening times, access to the shop, systems for dispensing prescriptions, etc. Relay any comments back to general practices if comments apply there. Listen to customers' views and act on them where appropriate.

Health promotion: volunteer that exercise is beneficial if asked to sell analgesics or NSAIDs for a 'bad back'. Be proactive with advice about the constipatory effects of some analgesics.

Risk management: identify risks of inadvertently dispensing the wrong drug and minimise them, e.g. doctors prescribing by phone, patients with same surname, deciphering GP's handwritten script.

Accountability and performance: keep records of monitoring systems and procedures to show good practice.

Core requirements: train staff so that they are competent to accept delegated roles.

Action plan

Agree who is involved/setting: as staff set out previously – specify names, posts.

Timetabled action:

start date:
by 2 months: preliminary data gathering and baseline of providers completed:

- is there a protocol for advising people with acute and chronic back pain in respect of self-care, medication, referral to others?
- range of medication and supportive equipment in stock, including complementary therapies.

by 4 months: review current performance:

- extent to which protocol or guide fits with best practice
- audit of actual performance via pre-agreed criteria – e.g. with respect to promotion of exercise and normal activities, level of medication recommended
- audit of significant event; for instance, patient suffering serious side effect such as haematemesis from NSAID.

by 6 months: identify solutions and associated training needs – plan learning activities and complete ongoing record of learning undertaken (*see* page 124):

- set up new systems for appropriate advice
- provide some in-house training to GPs and nurses in a multidisciplinary educational session.

by 9 months: make changes:

- regular patients to the pharmacy who are chronic back pain sufferers take more exercise and pursue normal activities.

Expected outcomes: more effective management of back pain; better patient compliance with exercise and attendance at referrals; less sickness absence due to back pain.

What additional resources will you require?

You may need funds for a patient information leaflet carrying the most up-to-date advice.

How much protected time will you allocate to undertaking the learning described in your plan?

That will depend on your circumstances, aspirations and needs.

How will you evaluate your learning plan?

You might re-audit any of the aspects of care and services that have featured so far.

How will you know when you have achieved your objectives?

Use the audit and survey methods described above and measure deviation from the agreed practice protocol.

How will you disseminate the learning from the plan to the rest of the practice team and patients? How will you sustain the new knowledge and skills?

Let all the staff know at practice meetings what progress has been made. You might want to describe your success at a PCG/T meeting.

How will you handle new learning requirements as they crop up?

Undertake an audit of the next significant event to find out whether the preceding care and services adhered to the practice protocol. If not, determine why not; and if so, what else should be changed or learnt?

Record of your personal learning about 'back pain'

You would add the date, length of time spent etc. on each learning activity

	Activity 1: becoming familiar with other providers who might help prevent or treat back pain	Activity 2: best practice in the management of back pain	Activity 3: update on medication relevant to back pain	Activity 4: learning about self-care of back pain
In-house formal learning	Physiotherapist, osteopath or chiropractor ran session for GPs, pharmacists, nurses and non-clinical staff in local practice	Local radiologist, pharmacist, orthopaedic consultant, community physiotherapist contributed to 'roadshow' held in practice for patients and staff	Pharmacist updated GPs at in-practice lunchtime session; pharmacist swotted up the latest recommendations about medication and side effects prior to giving update	Health promotion facilitator attended general medical practice and invited pharmacist. First planning meeting to set up 'exercise on prescription scheme'; plan talked through
External courses	GP and pharmacist attended update seminar on back pain that included review of what other health professionals can do	Pharmacist attended evening lecture at postgraduate centre on the management of back pain		
Informal and personal	GP and pharmacist pooled all literature together mapping out other providers – from Yellow Pages, unsolicited literature, from health promotion – over coffee	Pharmacist read through the patient literature left by health promotion facilitator advocating general exercises and normal activities for people with back pain	Discussed results of audit of anti-inflammatory drugs as practice team at meeting – invited pharmacist to join in	GPs and pharmacist chatted about introducing an exercise prescription referral scheme. Pharmacist visited health centre
Qualifications and/or experience gained	Certificate of attendance for course	Pharmacy extended range of treatments on offer by stocking TENS machines for sale and learning how they work	Retained audit and preparation notes in personal portfolio	Poster advertising scheme displayed in pharmacy; pharmacist able to explain the benefits and what it entails

Worked example 3: a personal development plan for a nurse or health visitor focusing on caring for his or her own and colleagues' backs

What topic: Back pain: in relation to manual handling and lifting.

Who chose topic? A nurse or health visitor working in a primary care setting might update their manual handling and lifting training if they have not undertaken updating during the last 12 months.

Justify why topic is a priority:

(i) *a practice and professional priority?* It is a requirement of the practice's or trust's Health and Safety at Work policy. Back injuries may be reduced if all staff are trained and updated regularly.

(ii) *a district or a national priority?* The most frequently given cause of a work-related back or limb problem by workers is manual handling, as described by 52% of those with a back problem. Using appropriate manual handling and lifting techniques will reduce the development of back pain.

Who will be included in the practice personal and professional development plan?

You might liaise with:

- GPs
- community physiotherapist
- local training and education providers.

Where are you now – baseline information?

This might include:

- whether you have a protocol for best practice in manual handling and lifting
- whether you know of providers of training and education that meet the requirements of mandatory training in this area, their availability and cost, etc.
- audit of the requirements of nursing and other work colleagues in

relation to whether they are up to date in manual handling and lifting techniques.

What information will you obtain about your learning needs?

You may undertake a significant event audit if you or a colleague have experienced a problem with manual handling or lifting, either within the practice or community setting.

You could undertake an audit of the next ten lifting episodes you undertake, identifying any risks and noting possible modifications either to equipment or your technique.

How do your learning needs match those of the practice as a whole?

You may find that your colleagues' needs are similar to your own in respect of their requirements for manual handling and lifting updating.

Patient or public input to your plan

As a nurse or health visitor you might ask patients to help you to reduce the risks from back injury, such as by positioning their leg in a certain way while undertaking a wound assessment and dressing, to help you to provide optimum care.

How will you prioritise your learning needs?

You only have a limited time to spend, so try to focus on issues where there are the maximum potential benefits for patient care.

Objectives of the PDP arising from the preliminary data-gathering exercise

To meet the objectives of the *Back in Work* initiative:[46]

- 'to reduce the misery and cost of back pain to those in the workplace'
- to 'promote good practice in back care management within a framework that includes prevention, assessment, treatment and rehabilitation'.

How you might integrate the 14 components of clinical governance into your personal development plan focusing on caring for your own back

Establishing a learning culture: discuss back pain at a regular meeting of the nursing team, which includes practice and attached staff; invite physiotherapist to join the meeting.

Managing resources and services: two nurses should be available to care for a heavy or awkward patient: it will be cost-effective overall to use two staff for one patient to prevent staff sickness absence if one nurse working on her/his own hurts her/his back.

Establishing a research and development culture: learn how others have devised and apply 'no lifting' techniques from reading published articles.

Reliable and accurate data: keep accurate and contemporaneous accident records in an official accident book.

Evidence-based practice and policy: include regular exercise in own lifestyle as preventive measure.

Confidentiality: keep information about other colleagues' health problems confidential, especially if they are patients of the practice.

Health gain: self-care of back with good posture and care with lifting.

Coherent team: all colleagues should be aware of lifting techniques so that one staff member does not cause a human weight or object to fall on another colleague unexpectedly.

Audit and evaluation: be able to undertake audit such as of a significant event if you or another colleague do hurt your back.

Meaningful involvement of patients and the public: involve patients in finding better ways to sit or lie or stand in their own homes that put less strain on your back and theirs.

Health promotion: include regular exercise in your own life.

Risk management: review any part of the job that is a potential hazard for your back. Use the risk assessments in Chapters 4 and 5 to look at your working environment at home, at work, in patients' homes; for example, your computer and workstation, or carrying equipment on home visits.

Accountability and performance: undertake regular audits to be able to demonstrate best practice; for example, completing an accident book, personal safety in practice or on home visits using check list in Chapter 5.

Core requirements: undertake training so that you are competent at manual handling.

Action plan

Agree who is involved/setting: e.g. practice nurse, health visitor, district nurse.

Timetabled action:

start date:
by 2 months: preliminary data gathering and baseline of providers completed:

- whether there is a policy for manual handling and lifting
- whether there is a system to monitor staff attendance at mandatory training sessions
- a list of who can provide education and training.

by 4 months: review current performance:

- audit to determine extent to which performance fits with best practice – lifting, equipment, calling for help, comfort in sitting at computer
- identify number of colleagues also needing updating in relation to manual handling and lifting over next 12 months.
- ask ten patients for feedback on being lifted.

by 6 months: identify solutions and associated training needs – plan learning activities and complete ongoing record of learning undertaken (*see* page 130):

- identify which organisation will provide multidisciplinary education and training relating to manual handling and lifting
- identify when and where training will take place and who will attend.

by 12 months: make changes:

- self and colleagues have incorporated new learning about manual handling and lifting in everyday practice
- a rolling programme of updating in relation to manual handling and lifting scheduled
- new equipment purchased to help lift safely
- taking regular exercise out of working hours.

Expected outcomes: More effective management of manual handling and lifting situations. Less back pain or back problems.

What additional resources will you require?

Apply to the practice manager or trust management for funding and time for the required education and training, and any necessary equipment.

How much protected time will you allocate to undertake the learning described in your plan?

That will depend on your circumstances, aspirations and needs.

How will you disseminate the learning from your plan and sustain the developments and new-found knowledge or skills?

Let all the staff know at practice meetings what progress has been made. You might want to describe your success at a PCG/T meeting.

How will you handle new learning requirements as they crop up?

Incorporate any new learning needs into the plan as it progresses.

How will you evaluate your learning plan?

You might re-audit any of the aspects of care and services that have featured so far.

How will you know when you have achieved your objectives?

Use audit and survey methods described above and measure deviation from the agreed practice protocol.

Record of your learning about 'back pain'

You would add the date, length of time spent etc. on each learning activity

	Activity 1: becoming familiar with other providers who might help prevent or treat back pain	Activity 2: best practice in the management of back pain	Activity 3: update on manual handling	Activity 4: learning about self-care of back pain
In-house formal learning	Section in community profile contains information on other providers in area who can help prevent or treat back pain	Local radiologist, pharmacist, orthopaedic consultant, community physiotherapist contributed to 'roadshow' held in practice for patients and staff	Physiotherapist updated GPs, nurses and health visitors and practice staff at in-practice lunchtime session on lifting and handling. Also watched video together	Health promotion facilitator attended GP practice with community nurses, health visitors and pharmacist, to plan 'exercise on prescription' scheme. Plan talked through
External course	GP, pharmacist, nurse and health visitor attended seminar on back pain including review of what other practitioners do		Those staff who have never had formal training in manual handling and lifting attended half-day course	
Informal and personal	GP, pharmacist, nursing and non-clinical staff read literature mapping out other providers – from community profile – over coffee break	Nurse reviewed patient literature advocating exercises and activities for people with back pain for readability, appropriateness and relevance to practice population	Results of audit of uptake of training relating to manual handling and lifting shared at next team meeting	GPs, nurses, health visitors and pharmacist chatted about introducing an exercise prescription referral scheme and advertising it in the practice
Qualifications and/or experience gained	Certificate of attendance at course	Range of appropriate patient literature increased	Critique of video and audit included in personal portfolio	Enrol self at local health club

Draw up and apply your practice personal and professional development plan focusing on health and safety (with respect to low back pain)

You will probably be interested in making the health and safety aspects of back pain a focus of your personal and professional development plan (PPDP) if you are a practice manager or a GP or pharmacist employer wanting to take care of your workforce and improve their working conditions.

Read through Worked example 4 on pages 137–145, which is a PPDP focused around the health and safety aspects of back pain. The example given is very comprehensive and you may not want to include so much in your own plan. You might include different topics and educational activities because your needs and circumstances are different from the example practitioner here.

Transfer the information about your learning needs from the reflection exercises at the end of Chapters 4 and 5 that you have completed so far to the empty template of the PPDP that follows. If you want to formulate a PDP focused on health and safety, use the template on pages 133–136, but consider it from a personal rather than a practice perspective.

Look at what you have recorded in the reflection exercises:

- Do you have policies in all the areas covered in Chapter 5?
- Do you manage the risks in those topics effectively?
- Do you comply with best practice in your policy on manual handling, personal safety, accident and injury reporting in line with RIDDOR?

- About ergonomics and posture.
- About health and safety.
- Measures in place for personal safety.
- In the risk assessment of your workplace and the tasks staff carry out.

The conclusions you have made at the end of each exercise will feature in the action plan of your PPDP. Some hints about transferring the information from your preliminary work are given in the boxes of the template that follows.

It might take around ten hours to draw up your learning plan, depending on what you do in the way of the preliminary needs assessment and the extent of learning and changes you undertake. The reflective exercises at the end of each chapter will fulfil most of your needs assessment – the time taken will depend on whether you undertake all the exercises or delegate them to a member of staff, or whether you are already performing well in these exercises. Incorporate learning about other important priority areas into your annual plan, too, – such as cancer, coronary heart disease, diabetes, etc.

Template for your practice personal and professional development plan[1]

Photocopy the four pages if you want to use the chart again for other topics

---

What topic?   Was it an individual or team choice?

Justify why topic is a priority: (It may be a critical incident, new government guidelines, special interest of team member, PCG/T urging you to adopt good employer practices that you mention here.)

a practice and professional priority? | e.g. Exercise 3 |
a district or a national priority?

Who will be included in the practice personal and professional development plan?
(Give posts and names of GPs or pharmacists, employed staff, attached staff, others from outside
the practice, patients or customers?) | e.g. Exercises 3 and 7 |

Who will collect the baseline information and how? Where are you now?
(You may choose to designate staff to carry out the exercises given in this book.)
| Selection of Exercises 1–16 |

What information will you obtain about individual learning wishes and needs?

Patient or public input to your plan
(You might ask a patient to note hazards in your practice or pharmacy.)

How will you prioritise everyone's needs in a fair and open way?
(Weigh the balance of the strategic or business needs of the practice and those of the staff.)

Aims of PPDP arising from the preliminary data gathering exercise
(So what exactly do you intend to do?)

How you might integrate the 14 components of clinical governance[3] into your PPDP focusing on the topic of health and safety or back pain in your practice or pharmacy
Transfer completed Exercise 1 or 2 from Chapter 1.

Establishing a learning culture:

Managing resources and services:

Establishing a research and development culture:

Reliable and accurate data:

Evidence-based practice and policy:

Confidentiality:

Health gain:

Coherent team:

Audit and evaluation:

Meaningful involvement of patients and the public:

Health promotion:

Risk management:

Accountability and performance:

Core requirements:

What additional resources will you require to execute your plan; from where will you obtain them?
(Will staff pay any course fees or undertake learning in their own time?)

How much protected time will you allocate to staff to undertake the learning described in your plan?

Action plan (include objectives, timetabled action, expected outcomes)
(Be specific. Draw on your conclusions that followed the audits and risk assessment. Be realistic about what you can achieve. Define outcomes now so that you can review what you have set out to achieve at a later date and know whether you have been successful and what else you should be planning to do.)

How will you evaluate your learning plan?
(Who will be responsible for what?)

How will you know when you have achieved your objectives?
(How will you measure success?)

How will you disseminate the learning from your plan and sustain the developments and new-found knowledge or skills?

How will you handle new learning requirements as they crop up?

Record of your learning about 'health and safety'
Write in topic, date, time spent, type of learning

	Activity 1	Activity 2	Activity 3	Activity 4
In-house formal learning				
External courses				
Informal and personal				
Qualifications and/or experience gained				

Worked example 4: a PPDP focusing on health and safety at work in the practice or pharmacy (with special emphasis on managing and preventing back pain and problems in employers and staff)

What topic? Health and safety at work in the practice or pharmacy

Who chose it? The practice manager suggested it. The practice manager might focus on it from a 'good employer' angle.

Justify why topic is a priority:

(i) *a practice priority?* Preventing back problems from manual handling by practice staff should reduce sickness absence. At present there are frequent breaches of health and safety law and no proper records are kept. A member of staff hurt her back pulling records out of a filing cabinet last month and is still off sick.

(ii) *a district priority?* The PCG has designated 'risk assessment' and 'risk management' as a priority for practices or pharmacies – in respect of health and safety and other clinical topics.

(iii) *a national priority?* The government *Back in Work* initiative aims to reduce sickness absence from back problems among the workforce, so retaining highly qualified or experienced members of staff in the workforce. Health and safety requirements are based on much national legislation.

Who will be included in your practice-based plan?

- all GPs or pharmacists
- practice manager or dispenser
- practice nurses
- reception staff or counter assistants
- cleaners
- attached staff who regularly use the practice premises – district nurses, community physio, health visitor, community midwives.

Who will collect the baseline information and how?

A practice manager or a GP/pharmacist employer might keep a prospective record of any staff member experiencing backache triggered or made worse by work. The practice manager or community physiotherapist could review the practice environment and watch people in their everyday work, looking for any causes of back problems that could be remedied.

The practice manager or a GP/pharmacist employer will find out which regulations relating to health and safety apply to the practice; who can offer help and advice – for example, any expert advisers at the health authority or local authority.

Undertake a needs assessment – how is the practice faring compared with what is required (for example, what policies are there, who knows about the policies, have any risk assessments been done in the previous two years?), identify gaps in compliance with the various regulations, extent of staff training, knowledge and skill base of the practice staff?

Where are you now?

Good employer practices – back problems in staff:

- is there a policy to minimise back problems in staff as part of an overall policy on health and safety or occupational care of staff? Are any measures in place to prevent back pain in staff? For example, has there been a training session on manual handling for all practice staff (including the cleaners) in the last year and, if so, who attended? Have sources of back problems for staff been reviewed (such as awkward filing cabinets; difficulties of getting heavy or disabled patients onto examination couches); and, if so, have measures been taken to minimise potential sources of back problems?
- are there any special sources of advice and help for staff with back problems? For example, special ergonomically designed chairs, advisory literature, fast-track to a physiotherapist?

Undertake a significant event audit of any recent breach in the law, or a patient or staff injury or accident, to see how systems and practices can be improved. For example, look at what happened when one of the district nurses hurt her back while on a home visit, lifting a patient who had fallen on the floor.

Visit another general practice or pharmacy that the PCG nominates as a shining example to see how your practice compares and pick up ideas for making improvements; adopt any of their policies and procedures that they are willing to share.

Include awareness/knowledge/skills about health and safety matters in each member of staff's annual appraisal, making training a priority in each individual's action plan as appropriate.

What information will you obtain about individual learning needs and wishes?

The practice manager or GP/pharmacist employer could put 'health and safety' or 'back pain in staff' on the agenda of the next staff meeting in the practice or pharmacy and invite comments and suggestions on improving health and safety at work – and volunteers to take responsibility for the various tasks.

What are the learning needs for your practice or pharmacy and how do they match the needs of the individual?

The practice manager or the GP/pharmacist employer should take a lead in ensuring that the practice or pharmacy improves the way it operates to prevent back problems in staff or to minimise the effects of back problems if staff are already sufferers. They would ensure that staff are trained in manual handling and know about back care. The GP/pharmacist will need to learn about the importance of investing in equipment and office furniture to minimise the risk of back problems occurring and join in any training on learning to lift in a trouble-free fashion or avoid lifting heavy weights altogether.

As the application of health and safety is a routine organisational issue, it is unlikely that individual members of staff will be clamouring to learn more about 'health and safety' for their own personal development. It is more likely that various staff will take on roles and responsibilities for the greater good of the practice in response to a direct request to do so.

Patient or public input to your plan

You might use patient feedback to identify problems in the practice that need to be rectified to prevent mishaps. For instance, a patient might tour the general medical practice or pharmacy to point out 'accidents waiting to happen' such as a trailing wire, torn carpet or hazards within reach of children.

You might have an 'expert' in your patient population whom you could invite to help assess your situation and suggest improvements – for instance, someone who specialises in ergonomically designed furniture.

How will you prioritise everyone's needs in a fair and open way?

In this instance the practice manager or GP/pharmacist employer should ensure that all the roles and responsibilities are allocated so that the regulations are fulfilled. It should be possible to decide for whom training is essential, for whom it is 'desirable' and who would like to attend out of interest rather than necessity. You might allocate the various duties at a staff meeting where health and safety is discussed; and the amount of education and training that is required by individual task-holders will follow.

Aims of PPDP arising from the preliminary data-gathering exercise

To increase the practice capability and expertise in health and safety matters such that you:

- comply with the regulations
- look after the wellbeing of the practice staff and promote fitness to work, particularly with regard to preventing or minimising back pain and problems
- maintain a safe working environment for staff and patients/ customers
- minimise the effects of work on the health of the members of staff.

How you might integrate the 14 components of clinical governance into your PPDP focusing on the aspects of back care relevant to health and safety at work in the practice

Establishing a learning culture: allocate roles and responsibilities for improving back care of staff in relation to health and safety; identify everyone's learning needs and arrange training.

Managing resources and services: determine what changes need to be made to the practice environment to prevent staff having to make awkward lifts or sit uncomfortably; invest in necessary equipment, training, etc.

Establishing a research and development culture: evaluate the effectiveness of a protocol to minimise lifting in the practice.

Reliable and accurate data: keep records of any back problems staff have at work – look for patterns and anticipate problems; keep accident and 'near miss' log book.

Evidence-based practice and policy: choose well-designed furniture on best evidence.

Confidentiality: tag records where patients present a risk to the health and safety of staff (e.g. of violence provoking back problems in staff); handle such information sensitively so that it is not released to anybody who does not have a 'need to know'.

Health gain: obvious health gains will result from, for instance, reducing or avoiding risks for staff from lifting.

Coherent team: the successful application of a health and safety policy in general practice relies on team members having a clear understanding of their roles and responsibilities.

Audit and evaluation: audit is an essential tool in monitoring standards of back care, in aspects of health and safety and in demonstrating effective risk management.

Meaningful involvement of patients and the public: a disabled patient might point out potential hazards for staff if he or she needed to be lifted, e.g. up on to an examination couch or when being fitted with an aid in a pharmacy.

Health promotion: promotion of good posture would have potential benefits for staff.

Risk management: training in manual handling techniques for everyone involved in lifting, however infrequently, should reduce risks of injury at work from lifting. New staff will need to be trained as part of their induction.

Accountability and performance: demonstrate that your environment is fit to practise from.

Core requirements: ensuring that staff are well-trained and work in a healthy and safe environment should be cost-effective, as mistakes and accidents are expensive if staff are affected.

Action plan

Agree who is involved/setting: as staff set out previously.

Timetabled action:

start date:
by 2 months: preliminary data gathering and collation of baseline of providers of advice/expertise, etc.:

- is there a practice protocol or guide on effective management of health and safety at work in the general practice or pharmacy; or other subsidiary protocols such as on personal safety?
- numbers of staff; map expertise; list other providers of advice/ expertise outside the practice or pharmacy
- information about past performance – recent audits or reports
- staff discussion to report problems that might trigger back pain and elicit their views and suggestions
- practice manager or GP/pharmacist employer observes people at work to detect potential sources of back problems.

by 4 months: review current performance:

- practice manager or GP/pharmacist employer reviews operation of services, e.g. are staff lifting as advised?
- practice manager or GP/pharmacist employer reviews extent of knowledge, skills and attitudes of staff with respect to lifting at work
- audit actual performance versus pre-agreed criteria, e.g. look at accident book – have all incidents resulted in preventive action and been followed up to check that changes are in place and working?
- compare performance with any or several of the 14 components of clinical governance, for example risk management and reliable and accurate data would be very relevant.

by 6 months: identify solutions and associated training needs – plan learning activities and completing ongoing record of learning undertaken (*see* page 145):

- set up new systems for reducing risks
- give practice team in-house training on important aspects of back care in relation to managing health and safety

- revise the practice protocols. Address identified gaps in procedures. Agree roles and responsibilities as a team for managing health and safety according to the protocol; certain staff attend external courses
- order new office furniture as necessary.

by 12 months: make changes:

- practice staff lift less heavy/awkward loads in better style
- clinicians adhere to practice protocol – as shown by repeat audits; staff feedback
- staff trained at external courses share knowledge with others in practice at in-house training session with external facilitator as necessary
- organise further training to anticipate new requirements.

Expected outcomes: better staff compliance with practice protocols on manual handling, health and safety; fewer or no accidents and injuries occurring in the general practice and pharmacy workplaces; staff wellbeing is promoted and seen as important.

How does your practice personal and professional development plan tie in with other strategic plans?

The practice's business plan and the PCG/T's Primary Care Investment Plan might both prioritise achieving higher and more consistent standards in health and safety in general practice and pharmacy workplaces.

What additional resources will you require?

You are likely to buy replacement office furniture and to fund that from the practice. The practice might pay for the course fees of any member of staff undertaking training that fulfils a priority need of the practice, in this case, health and safety.

Any learning cascaded to other members of the practice team as part of the PPDP should be undertaken in paid time and during working hours whenever possible.

How will you evaluate your PPDP?

The most appropriate methods of evaluation will depend on what specific aims you set for your PPDP; for example, if your main aim is that all staff lift safely, you might evaluate this by simply asking the community physiotherapist to observe staff at work. Or evaluate your achievements by assessing the staff themselves with a simple test of knowledge, or monitoring changes in practice.

You might undertake a survey of staff satisfaction with the new office furniture and their back comfort, before and after your initiative.

How will you know when you have achieved your objectives?

Record whether staff from different disciplines have taken part in the initiative, attended training on manual handling and put that learning into practice when lifting.

Usually this will be by comparing outcomes of your programme with baseline data. But it might also be determined by looking at staff compliance with the legal regulations as described in the practice protocol, or their levels of self-confidence in maintaining the aspects of health and safety for which they are responsible.

How will you disseminate the learning from the plan to the rest of the practice team and patients? How will you sustain the new knowledge and skills?

Let everyone know at staff meetings what progress has been made. You might want to describe your success at a PCG/T meeting or in a local report to the PCG/T. Review your practice or pharmacy protocols at set intervals to incorporate new information.

How will you handle new learning requirements as they crop up?

The practice manager or the GP/pharmacist employer might run audits at intervals and feed the results back to a staff meeting mid-way through the time period of the PPDP when there is time to revise the activities.

Record of your learning about back care aspects of health and safety at work

	Activity 1: application of back care aspects of health and safety policy	Activity 2: best practice in manual handling	Activity 3: improving personal safety
In-house formal learning	One-hour educational session facilitated by adviser on health and safety from local health promotion unit to all practice team; staff volunteered for various responsibilities	Community physiotherapist demonstrated best practice in lifting techniques and good practice at same one-hour educational session as for Activity 1	
External courses	Practice manager or GP/pharmacist employer attended day course at regional venue on legislation and effective management of health and safety in the NHS		GP/pharmacist attended local half-day course on improving personal safety
Informal and personal	GP/pharmacist chatted over coffee about implications of regulations whilst reading through the model health and safety policy, practice manager/senior staff member had drawn up	Staff looked at pictures of how to lift/sit pinned up on staff noticeboard. Physio toured surgery with GP advising on hazards and need for new equipment to reduce risks from lifting and poor posture	GP/pharmacist reviewed procedures to reduce risks to staff safety after course. Invested in better external lighting and alarms; new systems for keeping tabs on staff whereabouts
Qualifications and/or experience gained	Certificate of attendance at day course	Record of learning from own plan included in personal portfolio	PGEA accreditation for GP; certificate of attendance for pharmacist

References

1 Wakley G, Chambers R and Field S (2000) *Continuing Professional Development: making it happen.* Radcliffe Medical Press, Oxford.

2 Occupational Health Advisory Committee (2000) *Report and Recommendations on Improving Access to Occupational Health Support.* Health and Safety Commission, London.

3 Chambers R and Wakley G (2000) *Making Clinical Governance Work for You.* Radcliffe Medical Press, Oxford.

4 Lilley R (1999) *Making Sense of Clinical Governance* (2e). Radcliffe Medical Press, Oxford.

5 Royal College of General Practitioners (2000) *Access to General Practice Based Primary Care.* RCGP, London.

6 Dunning M, Abi-Aad G, Gilbert D *et al.* (1999) *Experience, Evidence and Everyday Practice.* King's Fund, London.

7 Chambers R (2000) *Involving Patients and the Public: how to do it better.* Radcliffe Medical Press, Oxford.

8 Department of Health (1997) *Report of the Review of Patient-identifiable Information.* In: The Caldicott Committee Report. Department of Health, London.

9 Donald P (2000) Promoting local ownership of guidelines. *Guide Pract.* **3**: 17.

10 Schers H, Braspenning J, Drijver M *et al.* (2000) Low back pain in general practice: reported management and reasons for not adhering to the guidelines in the Netherlands. *Br J Gen Pract.* **50**: 640–4.

11 Leboeuf-Yde C (1999) Smoking and low back pain. *Spine.* **24**(14): 1463–70.

12 Croft P, Papageorgiou A, Thomas E *et al.* (1999) *Spine.* **24**(15): 1556–61.

13 Garala M, Craig J and Lee J (1999) Reducing general practitioner referral for lumbar spine x-ray. *J Clin Gov.* **7**: 186–9.

14 Mohanna K and Chambers R (2001) *Risk Matters in Healthcare: communicating, explaining and managing risk.* Radcliffe Medical Press, Oxford.

15 Clinical Standards Advisory Group (1994) *Epidemiology Review: the epidemiology and cost of back pain.* The Stationery Office, London.

16 Clinical Standards Advisory Group (1994) *Back Pain.* The Stationery Office, London.

17 Government Statistical Service (1999) *The Prevalence of Back Pain in Great Britain in 1998.* The Stationery Office, London.

18 Palmer K, Walsh K, Bendall H *et al.* (2000) Back pain in Britain: comparison of two prevalence surveys at an interval of 10 years. *BMJ.* **320**: 1577–8.

19 Klaber-Moffett J, Richardson G, Sheldon T and Maynard A (1995) *Back Pain: its management and cost to society*. University of York, York.

20 Godlee F (2000) *Clinical Evidence* (June issue). BMJ Publishing Group, London.

21 Andersson G (1999) Epidemiological features of chronic low back pain. *Lancet*. **354**: 581–5.

22 Waddell G, McIntosh A, Hutchinson A *et al.* (1999) *Low Back Pain Evidence Review*. Royal College of General Practitioners, London.

23 Faculty of Occupational Medicine (2000) *Guidelines for the Management of Low Back Pain at Work*. FOM, London.

24 Thomas E, Silman A, Croft P *et al.* (1999) Predicting who develops chronic low back pain in primary care: a prospective study. *BMJ*. **318**: 1662–7.

25 Weatherell DJ, Ledingham JG and Warrell DA (1996) *Oxford Textbook of Medicine*. Oxford University Press, Oxford.

26 Royal College of Radiologists (1998) *Making the Best Use of a Department of Clinical Radiology*. RCR, London.

27 Silman A, Jayson M and Papageorgiou A (2000) Hospital referrals for low back pain: more coherence needed. *J Roy Soc Med*. **93**: 135–7.

28 Bonnet J (2000) *Complementary Medicine: information pack for primary care groups*. NHS Executive, London.

29 Ernst E (1998) Acupuncture for back pain. *Arch Intern Med*. **158**: 2235–41.

30 Meade TW, Dyer S, Browne W *et al.* (1990) Low back pain of mechanical origin: randomised comparison of chiropractic and hospital outpatient treatment. *BMJ*. **300**: 1431–7.

31 Moore A, McQuay H and Muir Gray JA (eds) (1997) Glucosamine and arthritis. *Bandolier*. **4**(12): 1–3.

32 Vickers A and Zollman C (1999) Herbal medicine: ABC of complementary medicine. *BMJ*. **319**: 1050–2.

33 Department of Social Security (1999) *Trainers' Notes and Visual Aids: medical training pack*. DSS, London.

34 Department of Social Security (2000) *Guidance for Doctors. 1B204 Guide*. DSS, London.

35 Chambers R (1999) *Survival Skills for GPs*. Radcliffe Medical Press, Oxford.

36 Roland M, Waddell G and Moffett J *et al.* (1997) *The Back Book*. The Stationery Office, London.

37 Howard N and Burn L (1999) *Alternative Answers to Back Problems*. Marshall, London.

38 Waddell G, Feder G and Lewis M (1997) Systematic reviews of bed rest and advice to stay active for acute low back pain. *Br J Gen Pract*. **47**: 647–52.

39 Health and Safety Executive (1999) *Good Health is Good Business: employer's guide* (MISC 130). HSE Books, Sudbury.

40 Health and Safety Executive (1998) *Five Steps to Successful Health and Safety Management*. HSE Books, Sudbury.

41 Chambers R, Moore S, Parker G and Slovak A (2001) *Occupational Health Matters in General Practice*. Radcliffe Medical Press, Oxford.

42 Health and Safety Executive (1998) *Self-reported Work-related Illness in 1995: results from a household survey.* HSE Books, Sudbury.

43 Dixon R, Lloyd B and Coleman S (1996) Defining and implementing a 'no lifting' standard. *Nursing Standard.* **10**(44): 33–6.

44 Home Office (1996) *British Crime Survey.* Home Office Research and Statistics Directorate, London.

45 Secretary of State for Education and Employment (1996) *Code of Practice of the Disability Discrimination Act 1995.* The Stationery Office, London.

46 Department of Health (2000) *Back in Work* campaign. Department of Health, London.

Relevant extracts from Health and Safety legislation

Health and Safety at Work etc. Act 1974 – extracts

Health and Safety at Work etc. Act 1974. London, HMSO.

s.2 'It shall be the duty of every employer to ensure, so far as is reasonably practicable, the health, safety and welfare at work of all his (or her) employees . . . '

s.3 'It shall be the duty of every employer to conduct his (or her) undertaking in such a way as to ensure, so far as is reasonably practicable, that persons not in his (or her) employment who may be affected thereby are not thereby exposed to risks to their health or safety . . . '

s.7 'It shall be the duty of every employee while at work . . . to take reasonable care for the health and safety of himself (or herself) and of other persons who may be affected by his (or her) acts or omissions at work . . . '

Management of Health and Safety at Work Regulations and Approved Code of Practice 1999 – extracts

Regulation 5 Health Surveillance:

'Every employer shall ensure that his (or her) employees are provided with such health surveillance as is appropriate having regard to the risks to their health and safety which are identified by the assessment.'

Health and Safety (Display Screen Equipment) Regulations and Approved Code of Practice 1992 – extracts

Regulation 5 Eye and eyesight:

'Where a person [is a user of display screen equipment] his (or her) employer shall ensure that he (or she) is provided with an appropriate eye and eyesight test, any such test to be carried out by a competent person . . . '

'Display screen equipment users are not obliged to have such tests performed, but where they choose to exercise their entitlement, employers should offer an examination by a registered ophthalmic optician, or a registered medical practitioner with suitable qualifications . . . All registered medical practitioners, including those in company occupational health departments, are entitled to carry out sight tests but normally only those with an ophthalmic qualification do so.'

The Reporting of Injuries, Diseases and Dangerous Occurrences Regulations (RIDDOR), 1995 – extracts

RIDDOR requires the reporting of work-related accidents, diseases and dangerous occurrences. It applies to all work activities, but not to all incidents. You (the employer) are required to report to the HSE or local authority if there is an accident at work and:

- your employee or a self-employed person working on your premises is killed, or a member of the public is killed or taken to hospital, or
- one of your employees or self-employed person working on your premises suffers an injury from an accident or an act of violence resulting in them being absent from (or unable to do) their normal work for more than three days including non-working days, or
- a doctor notifies you that your employee is suffering from a reportable work-related disease, or
- if something happens which does not result in a reportable injury, but which clearly could have done (a 'dangerous occurrence').

The terms 'major injury' and dangerous occurrence are defined in the guide to the regulations (*see* Appendix 2).

Sources of help

Websites

BackCare	www.backpain.org
British Acupuncture Council	www.acupuncture.org.uk
British Chiropractic Association	www.chiropractic-uk.co.uk
British Institute of Musculoskeletal Medicine	www.bimm.org.uk
British Society for Rheumatology	www.rheumatology.org.uk
Chartered Society of Physiotherapy	www.csphysio.org.uk
Chiropractor website	www.chirobase.org
Clinical Governance Research and Development	www.le.ac.uk/cgrdu/
Cochrane database	http://hiru.mcmaster.ca/cochrane/
DSS benefits	www.dss.gov.uk
Employment Services	www.dfee.gov.uk
European Agency for Safety and Health at Work	www.osha.eu.int
Health and Safety Executive	www.hse.gov.uk
Healthy Workplace Initiative	www.ohn.gov.uk
Institute for Complementary Medicine	http://www.icmedicine.co.uk
National Primary Care Research and Development	www.npcrdc.man.ac.uk
NHS Centre for Evidence-Based Medicine	http://cebm.jr2.ox.ac.uk
NHS Centre for Reviews and Dissemination	http://www.york.ac.uk/inst/crd
Oxford Pain Site	www.jr2.ox.ac.uk/bandolier/painres/painpag/index.html#Chronicle
Patient UK – info for non-medical people	www.patient.co.uk
Primary Care Learning Association	www.pcla.org.uk
Radcliffe Online	www.primarycareonline.co.uk
Royal College of General Practitioners	www.rcgp.org.uk
Osteopathic Information Service	www.osteopathy.org.uk
Trades Union Congress	www.tuc.org.uk

Organisations

BackCare, The National Organisation for Healthy Backs, 16 Elmtree Road, Teddington, Middlesex, TW11 8ST. Tel: 020 8977 5474; fax: 020 8943 5318; e-mail: back_pain@compuserve.com; website: www.backpain.org

British Complementary Medicine Association, Kensington House, 33 Imperial Square, Cheltenham, Gloucestershire GL50 1QZ. Tel: 01242 519911.

British Institute of Musculoskeletal Medicine, 34 The Avenue, Watford, Hertfordshire WD1 3NS. Tel: 01923 220999.

British Register of Complementary and Alternative Practitioners, PO Box 194, London SE16 1QZ. Tel: 0207 237 5165.

Chartered Society of Physiotherapy, 14 Bedford Row, London WC1R 4ED. Tel: 020 7306 6666.

Council for Complementary and Alternative Medicine, 63 Jeddo Road, London W12 9HQ. Tel: 020 8735 0632.

Faculty of Occupational Medicine, 6 St Andrew's Place, Regent's Park, London NW1 4LB. Tel: 020 7317 5890; website: www.facoccmed.ac.uk

Health and Safety Executive, Rose Court, 2 Southwark Bridge, London SE1 9HS. Website: www.hse.gov.uk

HSE enquiries: contact HSE's Infoline tel: 0541 545500; or write to HSE Information Centre, Broad Lane, Sheffield S3 7HQ. Fax: 0114 289 2333.

Institute for Complementary Medicine, PO Box 194, London SE16 7QZ. Tel: 020 7237 5165; website: www.icmedicine.co.uk

Society of Occupational Medicine, 6 St Andrew's Place, Regent's Park, London NW1 4LB. Tel: 020 7486 2641; website: www.som.org.uk

The Pain Relief Foundation, Pain Research Institute, Clinical Sciences Centre, University Hospital Aintree, Lower Lane, Fazakerley, Liverpool L9 7AL. Tel: 0151 523 1486; website: www.liv.ac.uk/pri/

Unison, 1 Mabledon Place, London WC1H 9AJ. Tel: 020 7388 2366; website: www.unison.org.uk

Complementary therapies

Acupuncture

British Acupuncture Council, 63 Jeddo Road, London W12 9HQ. Tel: 020 8735 0400.

British Medical Acupuncture Society, 12 Marbury House, Higher Whitley, Warrington, Cheshire WA4 4QW. Tel: 01925 730727; website: www.medical-acupuncture.co.uk

Aromatherapy

Aromatherapy Organisations Council, 3 Latymer Close, Braybrooke, Market Harborough, Leicester LE16 8LN. Tel: 01858 434242

Chiropractic

British Chiropractic Association, Blagrave House, 17 Blagrave Street, Reading RG1 1QB. Tel: 0118 950 5950; website: http://bca.chiropractic.org.uk/index.html

General Chiropractic Council, 344–354 Gray's Inn Road, London WC1X 8BP. Tel: 020 7713 5155; website: www.gcc-uk.org

Counselling

British Association of Counselling, 1 Regent Place, Rugby CV1 2PJ. Tel: 01788 550899; website: www.counselling.co.uk

Crystal therapy

Affiliation of Crystal Healing Organisations, 46 Lower Green Road, Esher, Surrey KT10 8HD. Tel: 020 8398 7252

International Association of Crystal Healing Therapists, PO Box 344, Manchester M60 2EZ. Tel: 01200 426061; website: www.iacht.co.uk

Herbal medicine

National Institute of Medical Herbalists, 56 Longbrook Street, Exeter EX4 6AH. Tel: 01392 426022; website: www.btinternet.com/~nimh/

Homeopathy

Faculty of Homeopathy, 15 Clerkenwell Close, London EC1R 0AA. Tel: 020 7566 7800. website: www.trusthomeopathy.org

Society of Homoeopaths, 4a Artizan Road, Northampton NN1 4HU. Tel: 01604 621400; website: www.homoeopathy-soh.uk

Hypnotherapy

The Association of Hypnotherapy Organisations The General Hypnotherapy Register, PO Box 204, Lymington SO41 6WP. Tel: 01590 683770; website: www.general-hypnotherapy-register.com

British Society of Medical and Dental Hypnosis, 17 Keppel View Road, Kimberworth, Rotherham S61 2AR. Tel: 01709 554558; website: www.bsmdh.demon.co.uk

Massage therapy

British Massage Therapy Council, Greenbank House, 65a Adelphi Street, Preston PR1 7BH. website: www.bmtc.co.uk

Meditation

Friends of the Western Buddhist Order, Birmingham Buddhist Centre, 11 Park Road, Moseley, Birmingham, West Midlands B13 8AB. Tel: 0121 449 5279; website: www.fwbo.org

Osteopathy

Osteopathic Information Service, Osteopathy House, 176 Tower Bridge Road, London SE1 3LU. Tel: 020 7357 6655; website: www.osteopathy.org.uk

British Osteopathic Association, Langham House East, Mill Street, Luton, Bedfordshire LU1 2NA. Tel: 01582 488455; website: www.osteopathy.org

Reflexology

British Reflexology Association, Monks Orchard, Whitbourne, Worcester WR6 5RB. Tel: 01886 821207; website: www.britreflex.co.uk

Association of Reflexologists, 27 Old Gloucester Street, London WC1N 3XX. Tel: 0870 567 3320; website: www.reflexology.org

Transcendental meditation

Transcendental Meditation, Beacon House, Willow Walk, Woodley Park, Skelmersdale, Lancashire WN8 6UR. Tel: 08705 143733; website: www.transcendental-meditation.org.uk

Yoga

British Wheel of Yoga, 25 Jermyn Street, Sleaford, Lincs NG34 7RU. Tel: 01529 306851; website: http://hometown.aol.com/wheelyoga

Bibliography

Further reading, books, journal papers, relevant reports

Chambers R, George V, McNeill A and Campbell I (1998) *Health at Work* in the general practice. *Br J Gen Pract*. **48**: 1501–4.

Cox RAF, Edwards FC and McCallum RI (eds) (2000) *Fitness for Work: the medical aspects* (3e). Oxford University Press, Oxford.

Department of Social Security (2000) *Medical Evidence for Statutory Sick Pay, Statutory Maternity Pay and Social Security Incapacity Benefit purposes: a guide for registered medical practitioners*. DSS, London.

Health Education Authority (1999) *Framework for Action: Health at Work in the NHS*. Health Education Authority, London.

Health and Safety Commission (1997) *Violence and Aggression to Staff in Health Services*. HSC, London.

Health and Safety Commission (1999) *Management of Health and Safety at Work: approved code of practice*. HSE, London.

Health and Safety Executive (1990) *A Guide to the Health and Safety at Work etc. Act 1974* (4e). HSE Books, Sudbury.

Health and Safety Executive (1994) *Five Steps to Risk Assessment*. HSE, Sudbury.

Health and Safety Executive (1994) *Getting to Grips with Manual Handling Problems* (INDG 143). HSE Books, Sudbury.

Health and Safety Executive (1996) *A Guide to the Health and Safety (Consultation with Employees) Regulations 1996*. HSE Books, Sudbury.

Health and Safety Executive (1999) *Essentials of Health and Safety at Work*. HSE Books, Sudbury.

Howard N and Burn L (1999) *Alternative Answers to Back Problems*. Marshall, London.

Jayson M (1999) *Understanding Back Pain*. Family Doctor Publications, Oxon.

Key S (2000) *Back Sufferers' Bible: you can treat your own back!* Vermilion, London.

Litchfield P (ed) (1995) *Health Risks to the Health Care Professional.* Royal College of Physicians, London.

Moore R and Moore S (2000) *Health and Safety at Work: guidance for general practitioners* (2e). Royal College of General Practitioners, London.

Royal College of Nursing (1995) *Health Assessment: advice for occupational health nurses.* RCN, London.

UNISON (1999) *The Health and Safety 'Six Pack.'* UNISON, London.

Waddell G, McIntosh A, Hutchinson A, Feder G and Lewis M (1999) *Low Back Pain Evidence Review.* Royal College of General Practitioners, London.

HSE leaflets

(See current catalogue. All HSE Books, Sudbury unless otherwise specified)

HSE leaflets, pamphlets and books may be obtained from booksellers or by mail order from: HSE Books, PO Box 1999, Sudbury, Suffolk CO10 2WA. Tel: 01787 88116/5; fax: 01787 313995.

HSE (1989) *Health and Safety Law: what you should know* (leaflet pack of 50).

HSE (1990) *First Aid at Work: Health and Safety (First Aid) Regulations 1981* (Approved Code of Practice) L 74.

HSE (1991) *Seating at Work* HSG 57.

HSE (1992) *Management of Health and Safety at Work* (Approved Code of Practice) L 21.

HSE (1998) *Safe Use of Work Equipment* (Approved Code of Practice and Guidance) L 22.

HSE (1998) *Manual Handling* (Guidance on Regulations) L 23.

HSE (1992) *Workplace Health, Safety and Welfare* (Approved Code of Practice) L 24.

HSE (1992) *Personal Protective Equipment at Work* (Guidance on Regulations) L 25.

HSE (1992) *Display Screen Equipment Work* (Guidance on Regulations) L 26.

HSE (1993) *Writing Your Health and Safety Policy Statement: a guide to preparing a safety policy statement for a small business.*

HSE (1993) *Your Work and Your Health: what your doctor needs to know* INDG 116.

HSE (1994) *VDUs: an easy guide to the regulations* HSG 90.

HSE (1995) *Health Risk Management: a practical guide for managers in small and medium sized enterprises* HSG 137.

HSE (1995) *Workplace Health, Safety and Welfare: a short guide* INDG 170.

HSE (1996) *Slips and Trips: guidance for employers on identifying hazards and controlling risks* HSG 155.

HSE (1997) *Successful Health and Safety Management* HSG 65.

The Disability Discrimination Act (1995). The Stationery Office, London.

HSE (1999) *A Guide to the Reporting of Injuries, Diseases and Dangerous Occurrences Regulations 1995 (revised)* L 73.

Patient information leaflet

You are free to photocopy the following pages for patients with back pain.

Back pain. What you can do to help yourself

Up-to-date advice based on current evidence, produced by the School of Health, Staffordshire University

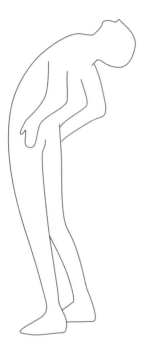

- Pain does not mean harm.

- Most back pain gets better with little or no medical treatment.

- Keep active, get back to normal activities as soon as possible.

- Build up your regular exercise to keep fit and prevent more back trouble in the future.

Most backache is not due to serious disease and usually settles fairly quickly. It can be extremely painful at first, and you may need to take things easy for a day or so, but resting for longer than this does more harm than good, as you can become stiff and weak, and feel even worse. It is best to try and keep as active and normal as possible, as this helps recovery. Getting back to work as soon as you can will generally speed up your improvement. Unless you are in a very heavy job, you don't have to wait until you are pain-free to start work.

Many people have back pain again from time to time, but in between are able to lead a normal life.

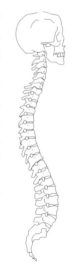

How does the spine work?

The spine consists of a column of bones called vertebrae, which are arranged as a series of curves, designed for strength and flexibility, supported by ligaments and muscles. It forms a protective cover for the nerves passing from the brain to the rest of the body, and between each bone, nerves emerge to supply muscles and to carry sensation to the brain. The lowest five bones make up the lumbar spine, and it is from here that the nerves to the legs are formed. Some of these join to make up a bundle of nerve fibres known as the sciatic nerve, which supplies the leg and foot; if this is irritated, the pain pattern in the leg is called 'sciatica'.

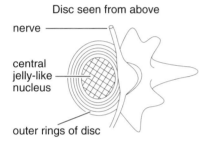

Disc seen from above

nerve

central jelly-like nucleus

outer rings of disc

Between the bones are discs, which cushion the spine from jarring, and enable movement even when weight is being carried. Discs are in two parts: a central jelly, which supports the weight, and a series of concentric rings which keep the jelly in place. Behind the disc is a notch through which the nerve passes, and behind this is a 'facet' joint, which allows movement of one bone on another. All the bones are joined together by ligaments. Occasionally a nerve can become trapped by part of the disc between the bones of the spine oozing out and squashing the nerve, or by a swelling in one of the small facet joints pressing on it. Sometimes being in a bent-forward posture for a long time or lifting with a bent

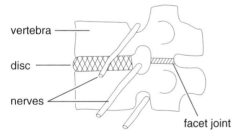

Side-view of two vertebrae

vertebra

disc

nerves

facet joint

back can cause the central jelly of the disc to move backwards as pressure is put on the front of the disc.

These problems usually get better on their own, but sometimes require a little help to get you

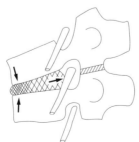

Bending forward puts pressure on the front of the disc

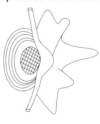

The nucleus shifts backwards and presses on the nerve

back to normal activities. Sometimes facet joints swell up and cause pain and locking of the back's movement. The main way of controlling this is to move as much as possible to prevent the spine seizing up, and to strengthen the muscular support for the spine, as it is often weakness of the muscles which aggravates facet joint problems. Even if the discs are worn and narrowed through 'wear and tear', it is important to keep moving to prevent the spine becoming stiffer and more painful.

Does pain mean damage to your spine? Not usually – most pain is due to strain of the ligaments and muscles around the spine, and these settle down fairly quickly. The strain can be the result of an accident, or can happen more slowly, through bad posture.

When people have pain, they often adopt pain-relieving postures, which can cause even more problems in the long term, as many ligaments and muscles shorten or lengthen to adapt to the new posture, and a minor backache can then develop into a long-standing problem.

There are **some serious problems** that your doctor can check out for you, but they are rare. You should see a doctor straight away: if your back pain is getting worse over a period of time for no apparent reason; if you feel generally unwell in addition to severe pain; if you have numbness around your back passage or genitals, difficulty passing urine, numbness, weakness or pins and needles in both legs, or unsteadiness on your feet.

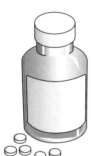

Most people do not need **tests or X-rays** for their back problems, and it is sensible to avoid unnecessary radiation.

To relieve pain, keep as mobile as possible and you should try to control your pain so that you can tolerate moving around. Remember that you are not causing damage to your back by keeping active. **Pain killers or anti-inflammatory tablets** from the pharmacist taken every 4–6 hours may be sufficient, or you may need to ask your doctor for something stronger if pain still prevents you moving about.

An **ice pack** (a bag of frozen peas wrapped in a damp tea-towel) placed on the painful area for 8–10 minutes may help to relieve the pain in the early stages, or try a hot water bottle or hot shower. A hot bath is not advisable as a treatment because the spine is in a rounded posture, which can aggravate the pain.

Keep a good upright **posture**, with a slight hollow in your low back, and when sitting, try a small cushion or foam roll in the hollow of your back.

Other treatments available are **complementary therapies**, which treat the person as a whole, and view your back pain as part of a wider picture of mechanical and psychological issues.

Acupuncture is effective in reducing some people's pain, and is especially helpful for long-standing back pain. Usually several – surprisingly painless – needles are used to stimulate a flow of energy (*chi*) to assist healing. Apart from acupuncturists with the qualifications MBAcC, many doctors, physiotherapists, and some osteopaths also offer acupuncture as part of their treatment.

Aromatherapy uses special oils to treat inflammation, muscle and joint pain, and these are sometimes combined with massage.

Homeopathy remedies are used in very dilute form to relieve different symptoms of back pain.

Hypnosis can help particularly where back pain results from muscle tension.

Manipulation can be helpful in reducing pain within the first six weeks, and can be done by chiropractors, osteopaths, physiotherapists or some doctors. Each will use different techniques, ranging from barely perceptible movements of small spinal joints to large forceful movements of the whole body. There is little risk with manipulation in the hands of a qualified practitioner.

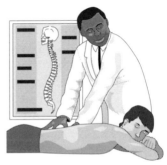

Massage is helpful for relaxation, but is unlikely to cure more complex problems.

Herbal remedies, either from Chinese or Western herbalists, are powerful medications; help should only be sought from qualified practitioners and treatment should be instead of, rather than in addition to, the use of conventional drugs from your doctor.

Reiki, reflexology, rolfing and shiatsu use massage techniques to move energy patterns in the body to heal pain in the spine and associated muscles and ligaments.

Relaxation can help to reduce muscle tension and mental stress, and this is likely to benefit recovery from back pain. Many complementary therapists use relaxation as part of their treatment, or you can purchase audio tapes that teach relaxation.

Exercise helps to prevent back pain by keeping you more supple, and promoting stronger bones and muscles, which give the spine more support. Chemicals released by doing exercise also make you feel better and reduce pain. Walking, swimming, cycling and rowing all help your suppleness, and at the same time make your heart and lungs work to improve your general fitness. Running can make the back more painful in the early stages of back pain, because of the jarring to the spine, so run on softer surfaces rather than roads.

> **Remember:**
>
> - keep active – bed rest is bad for your back
> - pain does not mean harm – it is quite difficult to damage your back
> - you may have good and bad days, but most back pain will recover quite quickly.

Other general exercises that can be helpful are yoga, T'ai chi, and Qigong. Although there is not a lot of

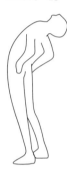

evidence at present to show that any one type of exercise is the answer for all back problems, some people do find particular movements helpful in reducing pain and strengthening the spine. Many physiotherapists recommend **self-manipulation exercises** which are described in Robin McKenzie's book *Treat Your Own Back*.[1] These need to be tailored to your problem, so seek advice. But basically, the kind of movement involved for reducing pain in the centre of your low back is to stand with your feet apart, and lean backwards ten times every hour or so.

This exercise may be done as a push-up on the floor instead, where you lie face down with your hands under your shoulders, and then push your arms straight, leaving your waist on the ground. For pain travelling down one

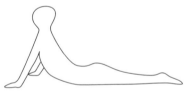

leg, a sideways movement compressing the painful side is used, often done while standing. Here, you stand sideways against a wall with the feet apart and the elbow next to the wall bent, with the painful side away from the wall; you then ease your hips towards the wall and then back to the centre again ten times. The pain should usually lessen or move upwards and towards the centre of the back.

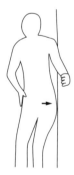

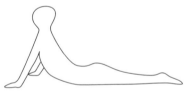

painful side

If this standing exercise doesn't help your pain, lie face down in the push-up position, but make a sideways kink in your spine with hips shifted **away from** the painful side, and do ten push-ups, leaving your hips on the floor.

Strengthening abdominal muscles is important for general support of the back, especially when bending forwards, when these muscles help to provide a kind of internal splint for the low back. It is better to strengthen muscles than use a corset.

Basic exercises are, briefly:

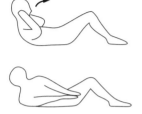

- lie on your back with knees bent, feet on the floor, lift head and shoulders off the floor, and reach towards your knees
- from the same starting position, reach one hand to the outside of the opposite leg, then change hands

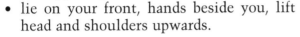

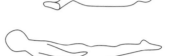

- lie on your side, lift the upper leg 30–50 cm
- lie on your front, hands beside you, lift head and shoulders upwards.

Do these movements slowly. Start by repeating them only a few times and gradually build up the number you can manage.

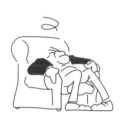

You must control your **posture** to reduce back pain and prevent further problems. The curves of your spine need to be kept as normal as possible.

Standing: the hollow in your low back often becomes flatter as you bring your arms forward to work at a workbench, desk or sink; put one foot on a small step or the bottom shelf of your base kitchen unit.

Sitting: slumping in an easy chair often causes the low back to become rounded. Put a small cushion or rolled-up towel in the hollow of your back to support it when sitting. With jobs such as using computers, machining or driving, it's the posture of the low back which is essential, as this is the foundation for posture of the other curves of the spine, so do use any adjustment in the seat or extra support like a rolled towel to help with your spinal posture. Move about every half-hour.

Ironing: adjust the height of your ironing board. Keep your weight evenly on both feet. Use a steam setting if you have one. Several short sessions are better than one long one.

Hoovering: get help to move large pieces of furniture. Don't twist your body. An upright cleaner means less bending than a cylinder.

Dusting/making beds/cleaning baths: kneel down to do these tasks, rather than bending your back.

Washing up: if your sink is too low, put an upturned bowl under your washing-up bowl. To keep your back straight, you can try opening the cupboard under the sink, and place one foot on the bottom shelf.

Gardening: kneel whenever possible – use a kneeler or knee pads. Don't jerk suddenly to pull plants out. Don't twist or strain. Interrupt heavy digging with lighter tasks. Use long-handled, lightweight tools. Several small loads are better than one large one.

Shopping: use a trolley rather than a basket, but make sure you haven't got the one with the stiff wheels, and be careful how you lift the goods out. Even out the load with two bags, one in each hand. Wearing high heels causes extra strain on joints by tipping you forwards.

Cleaning windows: use proper steps, don't stretch too far and remember that several short sessions are better than one long one.

Driving: if your hips are lower than your knees when sitting in your seat, try using a wedge or thin cushion to raise your bottom; keep a hollow in your back with a lumbar roll.

In bed: use a supportive, but not necessarily a very hard, mattress, or put a board under your present one, so that you don't sink into a rounded posture.

Lifting: this is much more of a problem when you have a 'bad back', and if you need to lift as part of your job, discuss with your employer whether you can be given some lighter work at first, so that you can start back to work as soon as possible.

Gradually, as you become stronger, you can return to more normal activities, and it is vital to remember the main rules for manual handling:

- Assess the situation: if you aren't confident that you can lift safely, get help.
- Be certain that the load is secure, you know where its central weight is, it isn't too heavy for you and you can grasp it securely.
- Make sure that there is enough space, the surface you are standing on is firm and you can avoid twisting where possible.
- Keep the load close in towards you.
- Keep your spine straight and lift the object by bending your knees and using your thigh muscles to do the work.

Make sure that you do not become overweight. Take regular exercise doing something that you enjoy, such as swimming or walking, for 20–30 minutes two or three times a week. Build up the amount of exercise gradually to keep the spinal muscles in shape.

Reference

1 McKenzie R (1998) *Treat Your Own Back*. Spinal Publications, New Zealand.

Index